Recognizing and Managing Children
with Fetal Alcohol Syndrome/
Fetal Alcohol Effects

Recognizing and Managing Children with Fetal Alcohol Syndrome/Fetal Alcohol Effects: A Guidebook

Brenda McCreight

CWLA Press • Washington, DC

CWLA Press is an imprint of the Child Welfare League of America. The Child Welfare League of America is the nation's oldest and largest membership-based child welfare organization. We are committed to engaging people everywhere in promoting the well-being of children, youth, and their families, and protecting every child from harm.

CHILD WELFARE LEAGUE OF AMERICA, INC.
HEADQUARTERS
440 First Street, NW, Third Floor, Washington, DC 20001-2085
E-mail: books@cwla.org

CURRENT PRINTING (last digit)
10 9 8 7 6 5 4 3 2

Cover by Sarah Knipschild
Text design by Jennifer M. Price

Printed in the United States of America

ISBN # 0–87868–607–X

Library of Congress Cataloging-in-Publication Data
McCreight, Brenda.
    Recognizing and managing children with fetal alcohol
  syndrome/fetal alcohol effects : a guidebook / by Brenda McCreight.
        p.   cm.
    Includes bibliographical references.
    ISBN 0-87868-607-X (pbk.)
    1. Children of prenatal alcohol abuse.   II. Title.
  RJ520.P74M33 1997   97-9039
  618.92'89--dc21

*T*his book is
dedicated to
Caryn and Jason.

Contents

Acknowledgments

As is the case with all books, this one could not have been written without the input and support of many people, including Pat Johnston, who helped me to change it from an academic paper to a book, and my editor, Carl Schoenberg, who did all the wonderful things that editors do. Dr. Basil Boulton helped enormously with his contributions to both the medical and psychological aspects of issue as well as his editing skills. It is important that I acknowledge and thank my grade 11 English teacher, Sue Hoffman, for trying to teach me to think, even though it has taken me 20 years since I last saw her to begin doing so. And, I want to thank all of the adoptive parents, biological parents, foster parents, and teachers who have been willing to share their stories with me, as well as all of the persons with FAS/E who have come forward at my workshops to tell me about their lives. I have tried to tell their stories as honestly as possible.

Introduction

This book begins with a medical, historical, and social review of Fetal Alcohol Syndrome and Fetal Alcohol Effects (FAS/E), followed by an overview of effective ways of helping and sources of assistance. The rest of the book is divided by the developmental stages of life from infancy to early adulthood. The different challenges and obstacles presented by the symptoms of FAS/E in each life stage are described, followed by suggestions to overcome these and to help the family, the teacher, and the child create effective changes in the child's behavior.

Nothing in the following pages offers a quick or simple solution, but the overall change in approach can result in a more hopeful outcome and can lead children with alcohol-related birth defects to an adulthood more successful than has been their lot in the past.

Throughout my first 10 years as a family counselor in a publicly funded agency, I kept coming across children for whom the standard methods of intervention repeatedly failed, regardless of the skills and commitment of the parents and the teachers involved. These children would frequently be diagnosed as "conduct disordered," and "borderline personality," or labelled as "budding sociopaths," or "children without a conscience."

As my first adopted child, Jason, began to grow, I saw many of these same confusing behaviors developing in him and so I began to search extensively for some other reason to explain why nothing that we tried worked with him or with the children on my caseload. I was spurred on to this search as I saw the emotional toll that the problems were taking on our own family, which at the time included our biological daughter, Caryn, and later included four more younger siblings, also adopted.

Since the years when Jason was a young child, the situation has changed, and the world is beginning to open up a little for persons with FAS/E. There is still much to learn, however, about how to help children with FAS/E increase the quality of their lives as they go through each day coping with alcohol-related birth defects.

I have written this book to provide others with the suggestions and general guidelines that I so badly needed when I was struggling to help my own son as well as the children and parents on my caseload.

Chapter 1
Our Story

The first time I saw Jason was at the preplacement visit in his foster home. The foster mother was caring for three of her own toddlers, two preschool nieces, and Jason, age 13 months. As I looked around the cramped one-bedroom basement suite, I tried to figure out which of the babies was to be ours. Suddenly, the foster mother handed one to me. I had him. In my arms. Our little boy.

The next few months were absorbed by doctors' appointments, infant development programs, and a bevy of specialists as everyone tried to figure out if Jason's obvious developmental delays were the result of neglect and malnutrition he had experienced while in foster care, or if there was some organic cause. His biological mother was known to be alcoholic, but he did not have the physiological indicators of fetal alcohol syndrome (FAS) so that factor was discounted and forgotten, as it would be by each of the psychologists and specialists from whom we spent a decade seeking help.

Jason gradually got stronger and he began to catch up physically to his age group. By the time he was two years old, he was moving and behaving like any other child of that age.

As time went on, however, it became apparent to us that some things about Jason were different. Our daughter Caryn was two and one-half years older than Jason and we noticed that he was not gaining an understanding of the world in the same way that she had. It was not the kind of thing one could put one's finger on. It was just that something was not right.

By the time Jason was four, it was clear that there was a problem. He could not remember colors, he had no sense of basic numbers, and he was still getting into the kind of trouble that children usually outgrow by that age. It seemed as if every rule had to be retaught every day and in every situation. Jason's speech was also a problem; nothing was clearly wrong, he simply made lots of little speech mistakes that the speech therapist was convinced would disappear with time.

As Jason grew, none of these problems actually went away. They just moved into different areas of his life so that everything Jason did was fraught with frustration on his part and on the part of the people who were around him. In Jason's earliest school years, it was obvious that he had disabilities in all areas of academic learning. It was also obvious that he had severe difficulties in learning simple games, acquiring new skills of any kind, or remembering the everyday rules at home and at school.

In my work as a family counselor I had frequently seen this same kind of behavior in the children, teens, and adults in my caseload. I had been taught, however, to attribute the negative behaviors of children to dysfunctional or ineffective parenting. Any thought that there might be an organic cause behind problem behaviors in children or teens was considered to be "victim blaming" and was discounted. Also, the nature of my caseload was such that alcoholism, sexual and/or physical abuse, and neglect were part of multigenerational patterns that would clearly lead to acting-out behaviors. A few families did not fit the stereotype of dysfunctional families, but they were a small enough minority that, with some emotional discomfort on my part, I could ignore the discrepancies between theory and the reality of these families.

So we muddled along. Jason kept getting into trouble everywhere he went; his father and I kept worrying and trying, and Jason's self-esteem kept plummeting. He knew he had problems and, according to his reasoning, if his mom and dad could not fix them, there must be something very bad about him.

Muddling along does not work forever, though, and one night, when Jason was about eleven, he and his older sister, Caryn, got into a normal sibling squabble that escalated until I felt I had to intervene. At that point, Jason, in a frenzy of frustration and anguish, grabbed and shook me. This stunned both of us. He was not a violent child and this behavior was completely out of character. When he turned and ran from the room, I ran after him and managed to catch him on the stairs. Jason sat down and started to cry. It was not a normal cry, it was a cry of the deepest despair I had ever heard. "Oh Mommy" he said, "I don't know what's wrong with me. I'm just an animal and I belong in a cage. Why don't you put me in a cage so I can't hurt anybody?"

There are truly no words to describe how I felt. If a heart really could break, I think mine would have broken at that moment. I did my best to reassure Jason that he did not belong in a cage, and we hugged and both promised to try harder. He would try harder to behave and I would try harder to understand. But we both knew that nothing would change and we were both afraid of what the future was going to bring.

From that point on I became desperate to find out how to help my son. Jason was a strong, kind, loving, wonderful child who had kept on trying to cope regardless of how he was treated by others and regardless of how confusing he found the world. But I knew that he was running out of steam and it was only a matter of time until he would give up. I was determined that I was not going to sit back and watch his life go badly just because nobody knew what was wrong. There had to be an answer and I was going to look until I found it. And I did.

Shortly after this incident, there was a segment on a television show about children who do not display all the physiological symptoms of fetal alcohol syndrome but still suffer some of the effects of maternal alcohol consumption during pregnancy. The children on the program had the same problems as Jason, and although none of them seemed to have been given a clear diagnosis of FAS, they were all being referred to as having fetal alcohol effects.

A book called *The Broken Cord,* by Michael Dorris, was mentioned during the program so I bought and read it.[1] The boy in the book suffered from symptoms that were more profound than those Jason experienced but many of the learning disabilities and the personality traits were the same. It was because Jason had close to normal intelligence and lacked the facial dysmorphology that the doctors had dismissed the idea of FAS in any form. And so that was it. I had the answer. We finally understood the problem.

As I began to understand the implications of this condition I realized how frequently it had been the underlying problem for so many of my clients. How many times had I decided that a family was unworkable when in reality, the lack of diagnosis of fetal alcohol syndrome/fetal alcohol effects (FAS/E), either in the parents or the children, meant that they were not being treated in a way that would work for them?

Unfortunately, none of the sources of information seemed to have many solutions or techniques or appropriate approaches, so Jason and I began to experiment with what helped to make his day go more smoothly and what did not. I stopped trying to change Jason and started changing my approach to the problems. I transferred our successes to my clients and combined what we were learning with the general information available on what was now being referred to under the umbrella term of alcohol-related birth defects. I then took that information to workshops where I was able to share my approach and to learn so much more from the many parents and caregivers who had been doing the same kind of experimenting in their families.

This book is the result of that experimenting and learning. It will not provide any quick and easy answers nor will it make the condition cease to exist. There are no happy-ever-afters for people with alcohol-related birth defects. I believe, however, that children with FAS/E can have a fulfilling and joy-filled childhood and go on to a productive and satisfying adulthood. The condition must be managed appropriately, and they cannot accomplish this alone, but with support from their families or caregivers, from the school system, and from anyone else with whom they have regular contact, they can do it.

Jason is now 17. He has good days and bad, and sometimes he still lies or steals, but mostly he does not, and it is never as bad as it used to be. In the last school year, he received three awards, two for being a helpful and cooperative student and one for being on the honor roll. He was also arrested once. But, he no longer perceives himself as an animal requiring a cage, in fact, he has a very healthy sense of self-esteem. Part of that is derived from his own feelings of successful management of this birth defect and the rest is derived from having friends, playing sports, and all of the same things as any other teen. When we think now of Jason's future, it is with excitement and hope and a firm belief that although life for Jason will always be a difficult challenge, it will be a challenge he can meet.

Notes

1. M. Dorris, *The Broken Cord* (New York: HarperPerennial, 1990).

Chapter 2
What Is It?

Alcohol-related birth defects (also known as ARBD) include physiological damage to the brain and body. The severity of the symptoms can be spread over a wide range and may be experienced through partial symptoms in one child or the full spectrum of symptoms in another. Children who display all of the symptoms, including prenatal and postnatal growth deficits, central nervous system dysfunction, specific facial characteristics, and body malformation problems are generally considered to have fetal alcohol syndrome. Those who display some, but not all, of these symptoms are considered to have fetal alcohol effects.[1] Fetal alcohol syndrome (FAS) includes the most preventable type of mental retardation with a prevalence of approximately one in 500 births. The prevalence of fetal alcohol effects (FAE) is not as well known due to a lack of recognition and diagnosis, but it may be as high as one in 30 births and, in communities with an unusually high rate of alcohol abuse, it may be one in five births.[2]

The people who suffer from this medical condition have an impact on a significant number of families, schools, judicial systems, and medical and mental health systems, yet services designed for their needs are almost nonexistent. Children with alcohol-related birth defects generally have both behavioral disorders and learning disabilities, but most educational systems are not designed to accommodate the two sets of problems when they occur in the same child. One child with this condition may be in a class for the behaviorally disordered while another may be in a class for the learning disabled. Where they are placed generally depends on the points of view of the placement advisors rather than on the needs of the individual child. To further complicate the matter, the children also have innate developmental needs that are often overlooked. In any event, it is difficult to follow a consistent approach to all of these children when so few are diagnosed.

People have probably been suffering from this birth defect ever since the first caveperson ate the first crop of fermented wild grapes. Society as a whole has not been any more willing to confront this condition than it has been to confront any other of the problems that arise from alcohol abuse. Society has known for centuries that maternal consumption of alcohol was directly related to problems in the offspring. An early reference to this can be found in Isaiah in the Bible, later references appear in early Greek literature and in the English Parliament in the 1800s; these references display a clear understanding that children born to alcoholic mothers were often physically or mentally challenged.[3] Society, however, has been entrenched in denial about many of the negative effects of alcohol and has only recently begun to pay attention to this particular condition.

In fact, it was not until 1973 that Dr. K. L. Jones and Dr. D. W. Smith published their studies of children born to alcoholic mothers and used the term fetal alcohol syndrome to categorize their observations. This condition is now the standard diagnosis for some of the birth defects that may result from prenatal exposure to alcohol. The term fetal alcohol effects was later used to connote a form of the same condition that manifested too few symptoms to fit the criteria for FAS.[4]

This understanding came about when researchers found that the impact of alcohol on the development of the body and the brain exists on a continuum, so that different combinations of factors may interrelate and cause differing degrees of organic dysfunction in different individuals.[5] In other words, at this time there is no way of making absolute predictions about how much alcohol consumed at any particular time in the pregnancy will affect the fetus, or which combination of factors will result in which problems. A study of alcoholic mothers published by Dr. Ann Pytkowicz Streissguth in 1980 revealed that one-half to one-third of the women who continued to drink heavily throughout their pregnancies had babies who fit the FAS/E diagnosis. This diagnosis is determined by observation of clinical symptoms that include: 1) growth deficiencies that are both prenatal and postnatal; 2) problems with the functioning of the central nervous system; 3) a particular pattern of facial characteristics.[6] According to Dr. Streissguth, many but not all children with what appear to be full FAS symptoms may also have an IQ in the severe to mildly retarded range and are generally hyperactive.[7]

The facial characteristics, or dysmorphology of FAS, allow for a fairly certain diagnosis. The characteristics include a short, upturned nose; a somewhat smaller than normal head; a broad flattened face with a wider than normal space between the eyes; ears a little bit lower on the head; a long, thin upper lip, and eyes with shorter slits.[8] A number of studies have indicated that some FAS victims suffer from heart defects and some may also experience kidney and urogenital tract problems.[9] As well, the ethanol component of alcohol targets the brain of the developing embryo or fetus and this invariably leads to later problems in learning and behavioral functioning. Skeletal abnormalities may also be observed and problems such as cleft palate and genitourinary malformations occur more frequently in children with FAS than in the general population. The diagnosis of the other forms of ARBD is less easily obtained. Individuals who have what may be considered as FAE may have growth or learning problems without any of the other symptoms.[10]

Because the FAE end of the birth defects spectrum is less clear than that of full FAS, and because it is more difficult to diagnose even when it is suspected, many children who have this condition are either not diagnosed at all or they are misdiagnosed as having a psychological condition such as "conduct disorder" or "borderline personality disorder." Still others are given a partial diagnosis of "attention deficit hyperactivity disorder" or "attachment disorder." Few of the individuals who have only one or two symptoms of FAS/E are appropriately diagnosed, and therefore many of these children are denied the kinds of supports and interventions that are effective for this condition. The tragedy is that these children are then inadequately educated and poorly socialized and so grow up to be at greater risk of becoming chronic welfare recipients, or substance abusers, or criminals. This is not because these behaviors are inherent characteristics of alcohol-related birth defects, but because these individuals have not had the opportunity to learn the social and academic skills that would allow them to live productive lifestyles.

The risk factor for development of alcohol-related birth defects is still not certain.[11] Some may develop a severe case, other infants who experienced the same amount of prenatal alcohol exposure may exhibit relatively minor symptoms. In fact, one study found a situation concerning twins where one twin had profound FAS while the other had only minor symptoms that would not likely have been noticed had the other twin not been so severely affected.[12] Any number of factors come into play in terms of risk for FAS/E, including maternal weight, fetal weight, cell development at the time of alcohol exposure, age of mother, overall health of mother, maternal use of cigarettes and/or other toxic substances, paternally derived factors, oxygen deprivation due to maternal liver dysfunction, genetic susceptibility, and other factors as yet undetermined by researchers.

Identification of alcohol addiction in the mother is also not a definitive risk factor. Women who have been identified as moderate drinkers have also given birth to infants with this type of birth defect. In fact, studies have shown that some women can drink heavily during pregnancy and produce a child who is free from this birth defect and others may drink minimally and produce a child who fits all the diagnostic criteria. The critical factor, or combination of factors, has yet to be determined.[13]

The ways in which alcohol affects the brain of the embryo or fetus are also still under study but it has been fairly well accepted that the ethanol in alcohol is the damaging factor in brain development.[14] Most of the studies have been done on animals but can be generalized to humans. According to one researcher, the ethanol acts by destroying cells in some parts of the brain during the early stages of the fetal development, and, in the later stages, it creates abnormalities in the ways in which the cells move and interconnect.

In other words, in the early stages of pregnancy the ethanol may kill developing and existing brain cells. In later stages, some brain cells may survive the toxic effects of the ethanol but will end up with disorganized cellular activity that results in learning disabilities and behavior disorders. Damage or disruption of the hormonal regulatory system may also cause later behavioral problems.[15] It must be remembered, however, that medical research on this problem is also in its early stages and new information and understanding may challenge or add to what is currently believed.

Notes

1. Dr. S. Clarren, "Recognition of fetal alcohol syndrome," *Journal of the American Medical Association*, 245(23), p. 2436.

2. Dr. C. Loock, *Prevention of alcohol-related birth defects fetal alcohol syndrome* (TRY, Alcohol and Drug Programs, Ministry of Health) p. 1.

3. *Ibid.*, p. 1.

4. A. Pytkowicz Streissguth, & R. LaDue, *Fetal alcohol, teratogenic causes of developmental disabilities* (work supported by Indian Health Service, the National Institute of Alcohol Abuse and Alcoholism, the University of Washington Alcohol and Drug Abuse Institute, and the Safeco Insurance Company, 1987), pp. 2, 15.

5. E. L. Abel, *Prenatal effect of alcohol* (a paper published by Elsivier Scientific Publishers Ireland, Ltd., Ireland, 1984), p. 2; J. R. West, "Fetal alcohol-induced brain damage and the problem of determining temporal vulnerability: A review," *Alcohol and Drug Research,* 7 (1987), pp. 423–441.

6. A. Pytkowicz Streissguth, R. LaDue, & S. P. Randals, *A manual on adolescents and adults with fetal alcohol syndrome with special reference to American Indians* (Seattle, WA: the Department of Psychiatry and Behavioral Sciences, the Child Development-Mental Retardation Center, and the Alcoholism and Drug Abuse Institute of the University of Washington, 1986), pp. 3, 6.

7. A. Pytkowicz Streissguth, & R. LaDue, "Psychological and behavioral effects in children prenatally exposed to alcohol," page 7, *Alcohol Health and Research World,* (1985, Fall), pp. 6–12.

8. B. Boulton, M.D., F.R.C.P.C., Victoria, B.C., Canada, 1995.

9. *Ibid.*

10. A. Pytkowicz Streissguth, & R. LaDue, "Psychological and behavioral effects in children prenatally exposed to alcohol," pp. 4–6, *Alcohol Health and Research World,* (1985, Fall), pp. 6–12; and *Fetal alcohol, teratogenic causes of developmental disabilities* (work supported by Indian Health Service, the National Institute of Alcohol Abuse and Alcoholism, the University of Washington Alcohol and Drug Abuse Institute, and the Safeco Insurance Company, 1987), p. 6.

11. J. R. West, "Fetal alcohol-induced brain damage and the problem of determining temporal vulnerability: A review," *Alcohol and Drug Research,* 7, p. 426.

12. E. L. Abel, *Prenatal effect of alcohol* (a paper published by Elsivier Scientific Publishers Ireland, Ltd., Ireland, 1984), p. 7.

13. *Ibid.*, pp. 7–8.

14. Dr. S. Clarren, "Recognition of fetal alcohol syndrome," *Journal of the American Medical Association, 245*(23), p. 2436.

15. A. Pytkowicz Streissguth, & R. LaDue, "Psychological and behavioral effects in children prenatally exposed to alcohol," pp. 4–6, *Alcohol Health and Research World,* (1985, Fall), pp. 6–12; and *Fetal alcohol, teratogenic causes of developmental disabilities* (work supported by Indian Health Service, the National Institute of Alcohol Abuse and Alcoholism, the University of Washington Alcohol and Drug Abuse Institute, and the Safeco Insurance Company, 1987), p. 6.

Chapter 3
Behavioral Characteristics

*T*he learning disabilities and behavioral disorders that occur with FAS/E are quite severe and have been documented by many researchers including those already mentioned in previous chapters. Although these learning and behavioral problems are always present they may go unnoticed until the child enters school. Sadly, parents and caregivers often dismiss the clues until they are confronted with definite problems.

For example, the stairs to our front door had two huge chrysanthemum plants growing beside them. One was yellow and one was purple and every time we walked past the plants, I would say the color of the flower to three-year-old Jason and he would repeat it. I had done this with Caryn and she had soon memorized the colors and generalized the label "yellow" or "purple" to other items of the same color. Jason, however, did not seem to be able to do that. Even more disturbing, he did not ever remember the colors and I had to teach him again every time we went up or down the stairs. I mentioned this to my husband and to other parents, and everyone seemed to think the same as I did, that he just was not interested in colors and would learn them when he was ready. By the time he was eight we were still waiting for him to be "ready."

In the behavioral arena, the same problems were occurring. We could never turn our backs on Jason, even as he got older, because there was no predicting what he would do. At the age of two, he might just sit and not move for half an hour at a time, or, in the time it took me to answer the phone, he might disappear out the door and I would find him climbing the rose trellis in the back garden. The common wisdom at that time was that Jason was "all boy," or, that he would "grow out of it." But we learned, over time, that there is no "growing out of it," only growing into more ways to make mistakes and more ways to get hurt.

Once the child enters school, the learning and behavioral problems become quite apparent as the normal social and academic expectations become, for the child with this condition, a setup for chronic failure and frustration.

The following compilation of behavioral characteristics encompasses those noted by the previously named authors and those characteristics I have observed in both my son and my clients. These characteristics are not part of a medical or psychological diagnosis, but rather they are a description of the behaviors. Many of these characteristics are common to other conditions or psychological profiles as well, but these characteristics differ in that they are consistent throughout the life of the individual and are not changed by regular types of counseling.

- Disabilities
  —academic
  —attention deficit disorder (with or without hyperactivity)
  —speech/language disorders
  —information processing deficit
  —patterning problems
- Poor impulse control
- Inability to relate behavior to consequences

- No sense of connection to societal rules
- Poor short-term memory
- Inconsistent knowledge base
- Poor personal boundaries
- Confusion under pressure
- Difficulty grasping abstract concepts
- Inability to manage anger (own or others)
- Poor judgment
- Tendency to be stubborn

This is a large list of things that can go wrong on any day. These characteristics make it incredibly hard for a person with alcohol-related birth defects to get through the day. Yet, because these people are so seldom diagnosed, most of the problems that arise from these disabilities are considered to be their own fault. In fact, the degree of emotional strength and persistence that alcohol-affected persons display is enormous. It is just that the rest of us do not know enough to recognize what is really going on and we fail to respect the struggle and courage it takes for them to keep on living.

Disabilities

Academic

Children with FAS/E often have a wide range of learning disabilities in all areas including language arts and mathematics, and they display difficulties using "executive functions." Muriel Lezak defines *executive functions* as having four parts: goal formation, planning, carrying out the goals, and doing so effectively.[1] Each has its own set of activities. In other words, if the teacher tells the children to get out their math books and do questions one to ten, each pupil must understand this in terms of first getting out the textbook, the exercise book, the pencil and eraser, and also clearing the desk of anything that is extraneous to the task or distracting. Then the pupil must understand the number of questions to be done in terms of a quantity with a beginning and an end, and, must make some judgment about how much time to spend on each question. After this, the pupil must begin the work, stay on task, use his or her knowledge of the subject, and finally, complete the task.

For most people, this process is not thought out consciously. The average pupil will simply take out the books and start working with only a few minor distractions from the task at hand. A pupil with this birth defect, however, is blocked at the start. The impaired executive function does not allow for the overall process to take place and the child's mind does not move easily into the simple beginning tasks of clearing the desk and getting out the right books. It is as if nothing kicks in to start the whole process.

Once the pupil does get started, usually after some prodding by the teacher, the ability to actually do the work may be blocked by the child's problems with dyslexia, aphasia, sequencing, spatial disorders, and so on. It is not uncommon for children with minimal alcohol-related birth defects to have just minimal learning disabilities. The disabilities, however, spread right across the learning spectrum, and a number of minimally disabled areas add up to a major gap in the ability to learn in general. Clearly, if every aspect of learning has some problem, no matter how small, then the general ability to learn will be severely affected and the child will miss most of what is being taught.

Attention Deficit Disorder

Attention deficit disorder is a common problem for children with FAS/E and, according to one expert, Dr. Russell Barkley, this condition can be differentiated into two forms.[2] One is the well known "hyperactive" type in which the child appears to be highly overactive and easily distracted, finds it hard to stay on task, and generally has a difficult time following the social rules. The other, according to Barkley, is called "undifferentiated." It is less well-known and is characterized by a child who frequently appears lost in a daydream, is slow-moving and looks unmotivated, and also finds it difficult to stay on task or to follow the social rules. The difference is that the hyperactive child is overstimulated by the outside world and the child with the undifferentiated disorder is overstimulated by the inner world, or, what is going on in his own mind.*

Lezak suggests that although "attention, concentration, and tracking can be differentiated theoretically, in practice they are difficult to separate."[3] In other words, these three parts of thinking may be separated into different categories in the textbooks, but they are all part of the same problem in terms of the child's behavior, because without the ability to pay attention, the child cannot possibly concentrate on, or follow through with, the task. Therefore, since children with attention deficit disorder cannot focus their attention for any significant length of time, they cannot concentrate on a task, and they cannot keep track of what is going on either externally or internally.

The difficulty with attention is not limited to learning situations or to school. It is a constant factor in the child's life and it interferes with the ability to play, to participate in team activities, and to comply with normal social expectations. The child with FAS/E cannot focus or concentrate on the unspoken rules of social and interpersonal relationships any more than he can pay attention to the clearly defined rules of the classroom or the algebra formula.

Speech/Language Disorders

In more cognitively handicapped individuals, speech problems may take the form of perseveration (repeating a word or phrase over and over), and repetitious use of phrases. Those with higher IQ scores may have problems with articulation, talking too quickly, interrupting, or mumbling.[4] They may also have problems with opposites, such as always saying "hot" when they mean "cold," or they may display speech patterns that

---

* The male gender will be used in this chapter for easier reading. Male and female gender will be used in alternating chapters throughout the book.

are consistently wrong, such as "That is the girl *what* came over to our house." These are common grammatical errors for all young children, but people with FAS/E do not always outgrow them.

Information Processing Deficit

This deficit is probably one of the most damaging for the person with alcohol-related birth defects because it permits the child to appear to be processing the information, thereby giving others an unrealistic expectation of what he will be able to do with the information. It is as if the brain's ability to connect the information with some kind of action is missing and information goes in the ears and out the mouth without any stops along the way. The child may be able to repeat everything that has been said, but the fact that the child can hear and repeat it does not mean he can figure out what to do with it.

One expert suggests that this deficit has three components: the "inability to translate information into appropriate action, failure to generalize information from one situation to another, and difficulty perceiving similarities and differences between events."[5] This means that even though the child is able to take the information in, he is unable to do anything with it. The information goes into the brain but does not get translated into a behavior or an action. Even if the child understands a rule for a particular situation, and manages to remember it, the child will not be able to perceive when the same rule should be used in a similar situation. He cannot tell what is the same and what is different.

For example, many of the these children appear to be addicted to sugar. Stealing food is a secondary characteristic and sugar items are the first to go. On one occasion, Jason ate an entire jar of Oreo cookies while I was out mowing the lawn. Needless to say, I was angry and I made sure he understood that he must never do that again! I could tell by the look on his face that Jason understood that rule perfectly. A few days later I refilled the cookie container with some oatmeal cookies. Sure enough, Jason got them all. In the process of trying to understand how he would deliberately disobey me so soon after the first incident, I realized that he truly did not see the similarity in what he had done. Jason had taken oatmeal cookies, not Oreo cookies, and as far as he was concerned he had not done anything wrong.

Patterning Problems

Patterning is a term that is used here to denote the ability to perceive the patterns, or common threads, the ways in which people relate to each other, the ways in which people relate to things, and the ways in which life is presented to us everyday. Most families have fairly similar relationship patterns in that there are one or two parents and some children who belong to those parents. Children with FAS/E are not always likely to notice or care about the fact that this is a common pattern for all the families they know.

For many years we lived next door to the same family, which consisted of Mrs. R (the mother and wife), Mr. R (the father and husband), and their children, Lisa and Jimmy. Jason would often refer to Mr. R as being Mrs. R's father rather than her husband. He also frequently forgot that Lisa and Jimmy were siblings and might refer to Lisa as if she were Jimmy's husband. Jason simply could not remember the labels that were attached to the roles, and could not see that our neighbors had the same pattern of relationships as our own family.

The routines that we establish to provide predictability and allow for organization in the home and classroom are also based on patterns that arise from daily living. The patterns involved in routine are invisible to these children and therefore, as one teacher said to me, every day of school is the first day. Very little knowledge of the routine is carried over from one situation to another and the patterns of life do not flow from one day to the next.

Poor Impulse Control

Poor impulse control is a direct result of attention deficit disorder, impaired executive functioning, information processing deficit, and poor personal boundaries. This frequently results in children putting themselves in dangerous or forbidden situations, as well as being one of the major reasons for stealing. Children with alcohol-related birth defects may see something they find interesting but they do not have the ability to stop and think about to whom it belongs, consider what he should or should not do with it, plan what he will do with it, or consider how others might react if it is gone. Before any conscious thought can occur, the interesting object has been picked up, pocketed, and forgotten as the children's' attention is diverted to something else.

Poor impulse control also leads to diminished attention span as the children flit from one activity to another depending on what has most recently caught their attention. The children may also exhibit inappropriate emotional states because the feeling that went with the impulse is forgotten before the behavior occurs. In other words, a child feels frustrated, experiences an impulse to throw a toy, but has moved on to a different feeling state before the toy hits the window. To the observing parent, there is no apparent link between the emotional state and the behavior.

The results of this in terms of rule-breaking at home and at school are quite obvious. In the larger community, however, the lack of an adequate attention span and lack of impulse control also make normal play and peer relationships quite difficult. The child with FAS/E frequently becomes confused during games or forgets the rules, and soon becomes alienated from the other children who need more dependability in their playmates.

Poor impulse control means that the child often lacks both the intent to commit the crime and the skill to cover it up, therefore, they generally get caught. Other children may also be stealing from the school or home, but it is the child with FAS/E who will be the most frequently punished.[6]

Inability to Relate Behavior to Consequences

It is difficult to understand a cause-and-effect relationship when you cannot always process the information that links the cause to the effect. The boy with alcohol-related birth defects, for example, may know that he just threw the baseball through your living room window but he may not understand just what that has to do with your being angry at him. To the child, this was an "accident" and therefore not his fault and not his responsibility to fix. All the factors that you, the adult, may be considering—cost, inconvenience, discomfort, and that you had also told him not to play ball near the living room window—will simply not be part of the child's understanding. You may discuss this with him until you are blue in the face, but if he is feeling confused or under pressure, he will not be able to process the information at the time.

This, of course, means that the type of natural or logical consequences used by many parents are of little value in terms of teaching the child personal responsibility or giving relevant punishment. There is no such thing as a relevant consequence to a child with this condition.

No Sense of Connection to Societal Rules

"Societal rules" may be considered to be those that generally require little teaching past early childhood because they are self-evident. For example, most children past the age of five or six are well aware that they are in danger of being hurt or killed if they run in front of a car, but children with FAS/E may be as likely to run in front of a car when they are 30 years old as they are at age three. This difficulty in absorbing societal rules may arise because children with FAS/E have a difficult time understanding how their behavior affects others or how they themselves are affected by things, events, or people. They fail to realize their vulnerability and frequently place themselves in dangerous situations.

When Jason was around 10 years old, we lived at the crest of a hill that ran down to a main city street. Jason liked to ride his skateboard down the hill because it gave him a wonderful opportunity to really get his speed up. Of course, he was not allowed to do that and he received many lectures on what could happen to him if he lost control and rode his skateboard into the traffic. One day, when I was driving home from work, Jason and his skateboard went whizzing past my car, right in the middle of the five o'clock traffic. My first thought was to make sure he was not hurt, and my second thought was to hurt him in revenge for his having scared me and for risking his life. Since I do not condone child abuse, I was prepared to replace an act of violence with the longest lecture he had ever heard (admittedly, this can be a form of abuse in itself).

Jason, however, was not responding to my yelling in his normal way. Instead of spacing out or looking away he just kept gazing at me with a funny half-smile on his face. Finally I could not take it any more and paused in my diatribe to ask him what he was smiling about. "Mom," he said, "you forgot to notice something. I can't get hurt because I'm wearing my bicycle helmet." We moved shortly after.

Poor Short-Term Memory

Memory has been defined as "the means by which an organism registers some previous exposure to an event or experience."[7] Children with FAS/E have memory, but they may not be able to recall a specific memory when they need it. This may also be connected with some of their other deficits because the child's focus of attention is constantly fluctuating and changing, and the information processing disorder prevents the brain from properly analyzing, channeling, and storing.

Poor short-term memory can lead to lying because the children, under pressure to come up with an answer, cannot recall what they did or did not do, and therefore give the first answer that comes to mind. And they keep doing so until the adult is satisfied and the pressure is removed. To the adult who wants an answer, this behavior appears to be deliberate lying. To the children with FAS/E, when the memory will not cooperate, there is no one answer that stands out as obviously true so any reply will do.

This also makes it extremely difficult for children who have FAS/E to learn from their own experience because they so frequently forget the behavior they displayed or the consequence that followed. And, of course, they will forget the link between the two. This often results in the same negative behaviors occurring repeatedly with little change or variation regardless of the way parents handle this behavior.

Inconsistent Knowledge Base

As discussed earlier, the ethanol content of alcohol targets the fetal brain cells and causes, among other things, disruptions in the migration of cells as the brain develops.[8] The resulting irregularity in the communications between neural systems causes the person with FAS/E to display sporadic and unpredictable performance throughout life. According to one expert, these are the children who know the entire alphabet one day, cannot recognize even one letter the next day, and three days later can print it without error.[9]

This presents confusing and conflicting behavior to a teacher or parent but the child cannot overcome such an obstacle without a degree of repetition and reteaching that is seldom available. The inconsistent knowledge base also includes rules in the home as well as in games and sports. Children who have FAS/E find it as difficult to retain consistent knowledge of the rules for soccer as they do for spelling. This means that they are frequently thrown off teams for cheating or disobeying the rules simply because what they understood of the game one day, they did not understand the next.

Poor Personal Boundaries

Boundaries have been described as "psychic bubbles which surround us."[10] The bubbles provide us with emotional protection and to prevent us from invading the personal space of others. Children with alcohol-related birth defects often appear to be lacking personal boundaries and do not always recognize them in others. This makes them appear very friendly and outgoing but it increases their vulnerability to exploitation and makes others uncomfortable with some of their behaviors. Streissguth states:

> This excessive friendliness is often combined with overly tactile behavior…Young children who are tactile are generally not considered deviant, but adolescents and adults who have little sense of personal space, are very "touchy", and have inappropriate and excessive curiosity are often disliked and shunned by their peer group.[11]

Streissguth also suggests that lack of boundaries may increase the likelihood that children or teens who are, or were, sexually abused, will act that abuse out on others.[12] In other words, they may be at risk of doing to younger children the same abusive things that were done to them. It is not that they are inherently deviant, but their lack of impulse control combined with lack of boundaries may lead the abused child to act out the trauma on other children without any real understanding of the impact of the behaviors. If a teen was a victim of abuse, lack of impulse control combined with lack of boundaries can lead a teen with FAS/E to go from first kiss to sexual intercourse without any intent to do so. The teen may end up feeling emotionally and sexually exploited even though he appeared to be engaging in consensual sex. This results in low self-esteem and confusion about how the teens see themselves in relation to sex and can often lead to a downward spiral of sexual acting out. In other words, the teens engage in sex against their own values simply because they did not stop to think. They feel bad about the behavior and about themselves and get a distorted and negative self-image. Further sexual behavior occurs because the teens feel trapped into the behavior of a sexually acting-out person.

For some, this may not lead to low self-esteem because of too many other problems with poor impulse control and an inability to consider consequences. In these situations, the young person may be sexually irresponsible and becomes at great risk of repeated pregnancies and of contracting and spreading sexually transmitted diseases.[13]

Poor personal boundaries also result in an increased tendency to steal because the alcohol-affected child does not have a sense of invading the personal space of others. One young teen, Linda, had a functional and loving family who had simply worn out from struggling through years of undiagnosed FAS/E-related behaviors. At the age of 16, Linda was placed in foster care with continued regular contact with parents. One of the parents' many concerns was their feeling as if they lived in a prison because all of their cupboards, closets, and bedrooms had to be locked in order to prevent Linda from going through them and taking whatever interested her. Linda was baffled about why this behavior bothered people. To her, she was always just looking for a sweater to borrow, or a piece of gum, or a quarter, or whatever she felt she was needing at the moment. She had never experienced the feeling of being intruded upon and so was at a complete loss to understand why her family was so distraught every time she "borrowed" something.

Confusion under Pressure

Taken in the context of all the previously discussed behavioral characteristics, it may be redundant to suggest that these children are easily confused under pressure. The behavior that so confuses and frustrates others is just as confusing and frustrating for the children. They must try to recall what has just occurred, try to understand why it is a problem for others, and then try to understand how to resolve the situation. This is generally quite overwhelming for most children with FAS/E and the only true answer they can come up with is "I don't know." Unfortunately, adults do not always perceive this as an acceptable response.

What the rest of us tend to forget is that alcohol-affected children are almost always under pressure of some kind. Their days do not go well and they know there is always trouble looming somewhere on the horizon. As well, it is not always possible for adults to recognize exactly what the children will interpret as pressure.

When Jason was about six, his aunt asked him what the color of his new bicycle was. He went quite pale and after a considerable period of silence, managed to stammer out the word "black." The truth was that the bike was red and that colors were still a problem for him. To his aunt, this was a simple question that she had asked just to get a conversation started. To Jason, this was an extremely threatening question that could only lead to problems.

Problems coping with pressure also mean that any new situation, with the inherent stresses and pressures that accompany a change in the routine or the rules, will bring about confusion and will make adapting to the changes very difficult. A move to a new neighborhood, a new teacher or a new classroom, creates enormous stress for the person with FAS/E and it may take weeks or even months of negative maladaptive behaviors before the child can find a way to fit into the new situation. These children do eventually adapt to change, but they require much time and support to do so.

Difficulty Grasping Abstract Concepts

Abstract concepts are ideas or things that change or shift, such as time and money. Both are perceived, valued, and defined in a variety of different ways. The constant change and invisible movement that is involved make them confusing for people with FAS/E. Time has almost no meaning for anybody who lives in the moment. For alcohol-affected persons, whatever they are doing at the moment is all-engrossing and any change in what is going on is dictated by internal or external stimulation, not by a clock. Since we cannot see time, there is nothing to give it meaning or to notice that it is in the process of passing. We may not actually see time passing, but we are constantly reminded in many ways that is passing or has passed.

Money presents the same problems. Streissguth reports that 95% of the people she studied could not handle money regardless of their background, age, or any other factor.[14] Inability to grasp abstract concepts (such as the relative worth of money) combined with a short attention span and poor impulse control make money a difficult concept for those with FAS/E, and it stays a problem throughout their lives. Problems managing an allowance at age ten will translate into problems managing the budget at age 30.

Problems managing money also contribute to stealing because the children do not grasp the value of money either for what it can buy or what it represents to others in terms of groceries, gas, lunch, and so on. Therefore, these children will, on impulse, take money from the parent's purse without any thought about how the loss of the money will impact on the parent. Also, the child will not likely understand why the parent gets angrier over a stolen twenty dollar bill than over a dime. They both have the same value to the child so the discrepancy in the parent's anger can be very confusing.

Inability to Manage Anger

The frustrations and constant negative interactions that are part of the daily lives of people who have FAS/E can become overwhelming at times and for some, the buildup of anger and the lack of impulse control may lead to a sudden outburst of physical aggression or an act of violence. Furthermore, many have experienced physical or sexual abuse that they may not have disclosed or may not have properly processed in therapy. For these victims, the lack of resolution of their abuse experience may also lead to violent acting-out behaviors.

People with FAS/E often appear to be as confused and frightened by their own behavior as the others involved in the conflict are. The inability to track and focus may mean that they cannot understand how they got to this point or how to get out of it. The anger of others toward alcohol-affected persons can also be frightening and confusing, as the children or teens may have no idea what they did to elicit this reaction. What is evident to the parent or teacher may be baffling to the children. They simply cannot make the connections that would explain why others are angry.

When alcohol-affected children reach their teens, anger management often becomes a particularly serious matter. Most teens, regardless of their overall abilities, have tempers and mood swings which are accepted as part of that life stage. Teens with FAS/E, however, are often denied their right to any anger because others confuse normal teenage anger with FAS/E symptomatology. As well, the adults involved may sometimes be less than perfect in the way they deal with their own anger toward the child. It is not unheard of in our home for me to be carried away with my frustration and anger at something Jason has done and to yell and generally mismanage my own emotional state. When I behave so poorly, I can justify it by saying that Jason pushed me too far that day. If Jason does the same thing, however, I blame him for not managing his anger appropriately.

Poor Judgment

Impulsivity, attention and information processing deficits, poor short-term memory, lack of boundaries, and inability to generalize, leave the person with FAS/E without the means to make appropriate choices or to use personal judgment. The first idea that is presented will be acted upon, the first suggestion given will be accepted, and the first choice is the only choice. Stopping to consider the alternatives, or to recall the rules governing a particular situation, is not part of the cognitive repertoire of choices available to the alcohol-affected person.

Since they cannot consider the consequences of any choice, persons with FAS/E are easily led by others and may become involved in break and enter situations simply because they were asked to join in by peers, not because they actually wanted to rob anyone. As well, because they make such poor choices in life, they often become scapegoats in the family, the school and the community.[15]

Giving children choices is a basic tenet of teaching personal responsibility, and most methods of discipline or education use the concept of choice extensively. For the child with FAS/E, however, use of choice is simply a setup for failure. The child did not really make a choice to begin with and, therefore, will not likely be able to follow through with the responsibilities that choosing entails. The result of the failure to follow through is generally a punishment because the child is considered to have broken his or her word, or betrayed your trust, or acted-out, when, really, all that happened was that the child had not really understood the implications of the so-called choice to begin with.

Cathy, a 16-year-old undiagnosed FAS/E person, was frequently truant from school. Every morning she became quite frustrated with her mother who kept nagging her about going to school and, of course, Cathy had every intention of going and staying there all day. Yes, she knew that she often did not do that, but that was before; of course she would go today. On the way to school, though, Cathy would run into a friend who was skipping and Cathy would tag along, or she would remember that someone had mentioned there was a bunch of whales out in the bay so she would just take a few extra minutes to see if they were still there.

The teachers were exasperated, the principal felt he had given her every chance, and she was finally told to make a choice. Either show up on time every day or be expelled. After all, she was taking up a seat in a limited alternative program and lots of kids who would make good use of the class were waiting to get in. Cathy knew that she had to get through school and she knew she was not ready to try to work so she "chose" to stop skipping. The next morning, Cathy listened attentively to her mother's warnings about what would happen if she did not follow through. After all, her mom reminded her, it was Cathy's choice to stay in school and so she was responsible for making it happen. Cathy agreed completely. In fact, she was almost at the school when she noticed a puppy that looked lost so Cathy decided she had better try to find the owner before the pound found the puppy. It took Cathy all morning but she did finally locate the owner, who was very grateful, and then she headed to school where she was promptly expelled for failing to follow through on her own choice.

Tendency to Be Stubborn

What we think of as stubbornness has been noted as a trait of people with FAS/E by experts as well as by anyone who has ever spent any time with them. This stubbornness is often very frustrating for teachers and parents because it appears to be just one more form of unreasonableness in such children's overall behavior. The reality, though, is that stubbornness often represents their inability to think clearly or to take in any more information at the moment. They reach a position of believing that they know something, and adding to or changing that knowledge is one step too many. They can usually move beyond the stubbornness if the adults involved are able to wait a bit and then try another means of providing the information.

Stubbornness can also become a means of control for some of these children. They have to live in a world that seems forever beyond their control, with apparently random rules and seemingly meaningless restrictions. Sticking to a position or idea or behavior, no matter how mad it makes other people, may be the only feeling of control the child or teen experiences that day or that week. It can be too threatening to let go of it for what appears to the child to be no reason at all.

Briggs, a noted author, links stubbornness with low self-esteem.[16] The author suggests that chronic low self-esteem results from feeling rejected and unlovable. As uncomfortable as this identity may be, it at least provides safety in its familiarity. When change is presented, the person feels threatened by the new demands and hangs on even tighter to the familiar, albeit ineffective, behaviors.[17]

This large list of characteristics is quite overwhelming to the individuals who have FAS/E and to others who try to relate to them. It means that almost every day there is some kind of problem, some kind of punishment, and some kind of frustration. Since the damage to the brain is there at birth, the characteristics are also present at that point and will be more evident as the demands on the individual increase with age. With proper diagnosis and appropriate intervention, these children can learn to cope with the condition and caregivers can help the children to lead a relatively normal life.

Notes

1. M. Lezak, *Neuropsychological assessment* (2nd ed.) (New York: Oxford University Press, 1983), p. 507.

2. R. Barkley, *Attention deficit hyperactivity disorder: A handbook for diagnosis and treatment* (New York: The Guilford Press, 1990) p. 184.

3. M. Lezak, *Neuropsychological assessment* (2nd ed.) (New York: Oxford University Press, 1983), p. 547.

4. A. Pytkowicz Streissguth, R. LaDue, & S. P. Randals, *A manual on adolescents and adults with fetal alcohol syndrome with special reference to American Indians*, (Seattle, WA: Department of Psychiatry and Behavioral Sciences, the Child Development-Mental Retardation Center, and the Alcoholism and Drug Abuse Institute of the University of Washington, 1986), p. 31.

5. B. A. Morse, *Information processing: A conceptual approach to understanding the behavioral disorders of fetal alcohol syndrome* (draft paper published by Boston University School of Medicine, Fetal Alcohol Education Programs, no date shown).

6. B. Boulton, M.D., F.R.C.P.C., Victoria, B.C., Canada, 1995.

7. M. Lezak, *Neuropsychological assessment* (2nd ed.) (New York: Oxford University Press, 1983), p. 414.

8. B. Boulton, M.D., F.R.C.P.C., Victoria, B.C., Canada, 1995.

9. B. A. Morse, *Information processing: A conceptual approach to understanding the behavioral disorders of fetal alcohol syndrome* (draft paper published by Boston University School of Medicine, Fetal Alcohol Education Program, no date shown) pp. 16–18.

10. S. Evans, *Shame, boundaries and dissociation in chemically dependent, abusive and incestuous families* (New York: Haworth Press, Inc., 1988).

11. A. Pytkowicz Streissguth, R. LaDue, & S. P. Randals, *A manual on adolescents and adults with fetal alcohol syndrome with special reference to American Indians*, (Seattle, WA: Department of Psychiatry and Behavioral Sciences, the Child Development-Mental Retardation Center, and the Alcoholism and Drug Abuse Institute of the University of Washington, 1986).

10. *Ibid.*

11. D. Corkville Briggs, *Your child's self-esteem* (New York: Doubleday, 1975), p. 34.

12. A. Pytkowicz Streissguth, R. LaDue, & S. P. Randals, *A manual on adolescents and adults with fetal alcohol syndrome with special reference to American Indians*, (Seattle, WA: Department of Psychiatry and Behavioral Sciences, the Child Development-Mental Retardation Center, and the Alcoholism and Drug Abuse Institute of the University of Washington, 1986).

13. B. Boulton, M.D., F.R.C.P.C., Victoria, B.C., Canada, 1995.

14. B. A. Morse, *Information processing: A conceptual approach to understanding the behavioral disorders of fetal alcohol syndrome* (draft paper published by Boston University School of Medicine, Fetal Alcohol Education Program, no date shown).

15. B. Boulton, M.D., F.R.C.P.C., Victoria, B.C., Canada, 1995.

16. D. Corkville Briggs, *Your child's self-esteem* (New York: Doubleday, 1975), p. 39.

17. D. Corkville Briggs, *Your child's self-esteem* (New York: Doubleday, 1975), p. 40.

Chapter 4
What to Do

At first glance it appears that the traditional intervention methods, such as using time out or logical consequences, have not worked with alcohol-affected people. It is not, however, the methods that have failed, it is the lack of flexibility and creativity in applying these methods to this group of people. Yet, despite years of documented failure, the same things are tried in the same way over and over, through failure after failure, suicide after suicide, prison sentence after prison sentence. Most of us complain about how stubborn and unreasonable people with FAS/E can be, and yet, professionals and parents alike have stubbornly clung to denial about the cause of the behaviors and have refused to try to change the way in which they approach the problems. Rather than accept and respect the realty that unalterable damage has occurred due to exposure of the fetal brain to alcohol, it is expected that these individuals will simply use willpower to overcome the disrupted and destroyed neural patterns.

Rudolph Dreikkurs, an expert on child-rearing, states that the goals of socializing the child to acceptable standards of behavior must be consistent, but the methods for doing so can change according to the changing needs of the child or the situation. Dreikkurs suggests that flexibility allows the parent to "influence" rather than change the child.[1] Dreikkur's advice is well-taken when we truly recognize that we are powerless to change the damaged brain function of the child with FAS/E, but we *can* influence how the child learns to manage the behavioral characteristics.

Children who have FAS/E are difficult to rear and difficult to teach. Difficult, but *not* impossible. The difficulties arise from a combination of the characteristics of the condition and from the emotional trauma that results when the characteristics prevent the normal, innate, developmental needs of the child from being met. If the characteristics are managed, or influenced effectively, the developmental needs will be met and the difficulties will be significantly reduced in the long run.

Three Steps to Intervention

Positive intervention has three steps. The first step is to recognize that FAS/E is a medical condition, just like diabetes or cerebral palsy, and must be treated with the same degree of respect. The second step is to involve alcohol-affected people in the management of their condition from the earliest possible age. It is disrespectful to exclude them from the knowledge of their diagnosis, and they should be an active part of the successful management of the characteristics. The third step is to throw out or alter any counseling and intervention approaches that have previously failed and start experimenting with methods that are suitable to the specific characteristics of the condition.

FAS/E as a Medical Condition

Alcoholism, especially in women, has generally gone hand in hand with both shame and denial. The shame becomes an inherent part of alcoholics' personalities as they experience their own negative judgment and that of others. The denial

often comes in the form of pretending someone is not alcoholic and by ignoring the negative consequences of the emotional chaos and family dysfunction that spin off from the alcoholic behavior. Somehow, the shame and denial that society loads onto alcoholics have oozed onto alcohol-affected
persons. They are blamed and shamed for the characteristics
and are held responsible for the problems in their lives.

For centuries it has been known that excessive maternal
drinking creates problems in the offspring, yet medical science
did not even have a name for the condition until 20 years ago.
Society has denied the reality of the condition and we have
denied any responsibility for the daily trauma that is part of
the life of an alcohol-affected child or adult. Instead of recognizing the cause of the problems and creating educational and
social support systems to alleviate them, society has continued to blame the individuals and punish them for failing to
change. No one would ever ask a child who was diagnosed
with severe cerebral palsy to run three laps around the gym-
nasium, but few us hesitate to ask a child with FAS/E to just
sit down and behave. We recognize and respect the needs of
the child with the visible handicap while completely rejecting
the equally valid needs of the child with this particular type of
birth defect.

It is common in schools today to see special devices on the
stairways that enable children in wheelchairs to have easy
access to classrooms on every floor of the school. It is also
common to see special textbooks designed for the sight-impaired and to see aides assigned to assist children with serious
physical challenges. One seldom, if ever, sees teacher's aides
assigned to children with FAS/E or textbooks designed for the
different learning needs of these children. Just as the child
with visible handicaps requires certain supports to obtain an
education so does the child with FAS/E. Yet, children with
this condition are often denied their right to an education due
to the lack of diagnosis and concurrent lack of supports. This
lack of respect and support will continue until society as a

whole can learn and accept that certain negative behaviors are characteristic of a medical condition resulting from prenatal exposure to alcohol. It is a birth defect; it is a medical condition; it is *not* a bad attitude.

People with FAS/E are often blamed for their negative behaviors, but frequently they are not given enough information about the condition to take any responsibility for appropriate change. I have had many parents in my office who have been adamant that they do not want their adopted child to know that he or she may have FAS/E. In these situations, the parents, teachers, and counselors may attend meetings and discuss the needs of the child in terms of the diagnosis, but the child is not given the same information and is then blamed when she or he does not actively participate in the planned change.

Some of the adoptive parents were unwilling to tell the child the truth because they were afraid of how the child would receive the information. They perceived withholding the information as a form of protection for the child. In reality, however, this is another form of denial that prevents positive change. Other adoptive parents have also refused to tell their child because they possess values that link alcoholism with shame. These parents view the condition of FAS/E as shameful, and they do not want their friends to find out that their child has been tainted by alcoholism. Clearly, in these families, the children have little chance for positive change or for developing self-esteem until the parents have worked through their own negative attitudes.

Some biological parents are overwhelmed by the guilt they feel about creating the condition in their child. But successful parenting is not based on guilt and it is important that these parents deal with their guilt and face the child honestly. Most children do very well with the truth and can appreciate the sincerity of their parents' sorrow over the unchangeable past. As well, until recently, most parents did not know that the alcohol that was consumed during pregnancy could create permanent damage in the child. These mothers usually assumed that even if the baby got drunk from the alcohol, it would "sober up." The information we have available today was not available for most women in the past and even now, many still do not have a complete understanding of how devastating this problem can be.

If the persons who are explaining the diagnosis to these children have a positive attitude about it, so will the children. They may go through stages of healthy anger and grief but they will resolve the feelings and will be able to accept the challenge of positive change. Many of the teens with whom I have worked were convinced they were either crazy or evil, but when they learned that their problems were the result of a medical condition they experienced emotional relief, and more importantly, hope.

It is best if the child simply grows up knowing that he or she has FAS/E. The parents can provide the information according to the child's developmental stage and ability to understand why some limitations or expectations exist in his or life. Some children will not be diagnosed until they are older, or even until adulthood, but as soon as the parents learn of the condition, the child, teen, or adult should also be informed.

At one of my workshops, a 32-year-old man, whom I will name Mr. L, came up to me and told me that he had spent the last ten years of his life as an alcoholic on the streets of downtown Vancouver. He had grown up believing he was bad and could never have a future, so he had given up on himself long before he was out of his teens. The turnaround came when his mother, who had never given up on him, attended one of my workshops and recognized that her son possessed FAS/E characteristics. She sought her son and convinced him to have her suspicions confirmed by a physician. After he received the definite diagnosis of FAE, Mr. L decided to give life another try. He underwent treatment for drug and alcohol abuse, got into a job training program, and within a year he was sober and earning a paycheck for the first time in his life.

The reason Mr. L was so successful was because he had a family with unusual strength, compassion, and resilience. They were still willing to give him the support and encouragement he needed to make one last try. Without knowing what his problem was, however, he might not have made that last attempt at sobriety and life.

Self-Management

Children and teens who have FAS/E do not readily respond to the traditional behavioral approaches because they usually cannot learn to manage their behaviors in the amount of time they are given before being declared unworkable. The lack of response to most treatments occurs for two reasons. First, most traditional methods of behavioral intervention are based on assumptions that the children or teens have age appropriate impulse control, that they can always understand how to perform the behaviors that are required, and that they will learn from experience. None of these assumptions is true for alcohol-affected persons. The second problem is that the traditional approaches are used in ways that are too limited in scope and too short-term to have any lasting affect. Residential programs often expel or discharge teens who fail to obey curfews, yet one of the characteristics of FAS/E is an inability to link behaviors with consequences. It is reasonable to expect that FAS/E teens will fail to show up on time for the first few weeks, or even months. These children also lie and steal because of the poor impulse control and an inconsistent knowledge base. After the second or third theft, many group home parents feel they have no choice but to terminate their contract in order to keep the possessions of the other residents safe.

Many schools provide support for the behaviorally disturbed and the learning-disabled. Children with alcohol-related birth defects generally end up in one of these two programs, leaving the other side of their disorders unattended. As well, children who have behavior problems due to external traumas such as sexual abuse or alcoholic parents, require and respond to different forms of behavior management techniques than children with an internal trauma such as FAS/E.

Many school administrations believe in fully mainstreaming behaviorally disordered children before the children show any signs of being able to cope in the regular classroom regardless of the support provided. If the children are not able to cope with the stimulation and rules of the classroom, they will invariably act out their distress by displaying negative behaviors. Under these conditions, neither the alcohol-affected child nor the rest of the children in the class have any opportunity to learn anything. The alcohol-affected children are expected to overcome the characteristics of FAS/E without any of the necessary supports and conditions available for them to do so.

Children with FAS/E have the need to develop physically, emotionally, intellectually, sexually, and spiritually just like any other child. They will, however, be hampered in their ability to proceed through the developmental stages of life by the level of their intelligence and by the characteristics of FAS/E. The IQ levels in children with alcohol related birth defects range from severely retarded to highly intelligent and each child must be taught how to deal with the characteristics at a level that is appropriate to his or her cognitive abilities.

Individualized, Flexible Helping

There is no single approach that will work for all people with FAS/E and there is no single approach that will work all the time for the same person. Helping children learn to manage their difficulties requires that the parents, the teachers, caregivers, and the counselors use creativity, consistency, reinforcement, time, and compassion.

Creativity is important in responding to the child's need for effective discipline. Since children with FAS/E have trouble relating a behavior to its consequences, the parents are continually challenged to use various ways of helping their children see the links between behavior and consequences, often virtually inventing methods of intervention that will have some impact, or influence, on the child's behavior. She or he must learn limits and boundaries, but since the child will not likely learn them through role modeling or observing daily life, new and dynamic means must be found. Instead of giving up when something either does not work immediately or ceases to work after a few weeks, the parents must have faith that something will eventually work and they must keep trying until the right method is found.

Children with FAS/E appear to lack an internal structure that allows them to perceive boundaries, patterns, and sequences. Consistency provides that structure in an external form so that it can be imposed over the child's life until such time when the child is able to incorporate those parts of human behavior and relationships into his or her own worldview.

Reinforcement means a constant reteaching of everything that the child is expected to understand about the world, including relationships and expectations. It is a partner to consistency and helps to override the problems arising from an inconsistent knowledge base and poor judgment. The academic and behavioral expectations will be more in line with the child's actual ability when there is an assumption that most things will have to be relearned and reinforced regularly. Reinforcement also decreases the setup for failure and low self-esteem that occurs when the adults assume that the child should know from previous experience how to behave in a particular situation.

The time it takes to be effective with a child with FAS/E is much greater than most people expect. Creativity, consistency, and reinforcement must be used for years. The goals for behavioral change are always long-term, and outcomes, such as learning to understand personal boundaries, are always planned in terms of when the child reaches adulthood. If the child is able to attain some of the goals earlier, then accept it as a wonderful bonus, not as the norm or as the new standard. The more dysfunctional or traumatic the child's life is, the more time everything will take. A child from a safe and nurturing environment may be fairly responsible about curfews by the time she or he reaches the middle teen years. A child whose energy has gone into surviving the chaos of a violent or alcoholic home will not likely respond to any curfews. The parents cannot successfully impose limits on the amount of time it will take the child to learn to manage FAS/E.

Compassion for the child is vital but it can become lost in the day-to-day problems, struggles, failures, and misbehaviors. One particularly bad spring, when Jason was 13, I was receiving calls from his school principal every day. She was irate, frustrated, and just plain tired of dealing with him, and I was feeling the same way. The stress was beginning to take its toll on my job performance, and it had reduced my ability to cope with the less severe (but equally important) problems of my other children. I resented the emotional energy Jason was taking from me and we were all basically fed up with him. Of course, this attitude on our part led to an escalation of his behaviors. The spiral seemed to be going on without an end in sight.

It all culminated one day when I received a call from the principal at nine o'clock in the morning informing me that Jason had pulled one stunt too many and they had decided to expel him from school. The principal had told Jason to leave, and he stormed off. No one knew where he had gone, and by this point, I suppose, they did not really care. We live in a small community, however, that is a one-hour bus ride from the location of his school near the downtown area of the city. I knew Jason would be caught up with feelings of anger toward the principal and fear of how I would react, and I was afraid of what he might do. To top it all off, this was happening around the first anniversary of his father's death from cancer, and Jason had recently been going through a period of being fascinated with death. Because I was terrified that he might either try to kill himself or might place himself in a risky situation, I was finally able to look at how the last few weeks must have been for Jason and I could, at last, feel compassion for what he had been going through.

I waited a few hours to see if he would arrive off the bus, but when he was not home for supper, I called the police. They were very kind and went and looked at a beach he used to go to with his dad, as well as a few of the teen hangouts in town. But there was no sign of him. After a while I did what I always do when he is out and I am afraid for him. I went into his bedroom and started cleaning. I do not know why I do this but this ritual began when he was little and, for some reason, I find it comforting. When I opened his closet door to hang up a shirt, there was Jason. He was curled up on the floor of his closet, wrapped in a blanket and sound asleep. I stroked his cheek and he woke up. "Hi, mom" he said, "I've had a hard day." So few words for so much pain. I realized that although he had been behaving badly for weeks (stealing, lying, acting aggressively), there had been no time at which either the principal or I had stopped to consider how his behavior must have felt to him. He had deserved the consequences that he had been receiving, and he did have to learn to manage some of his behaviors better, but we could have provided all of the same methods of discipline with some degree of overt compassion for him. We had not, and we had pushed Jason to the point that his only safety and comfort was in the back of a closet in a fetal position.

The need for parental creativity, consistency, reinforcement, time, and compassion exist in all children. Children with FAS/E need these forms of support more frequently and show less immediate reward to those who are doing the giving. It can feel as if the children take and take and take with little positive change to show for all of the effort. All those involved with children with FAS/E must learn to focus on the smallest of improvements, and to see their intervention as part of a long-term investment in the child with payoffs that the adult may not be around to see, like particular teachers or child care workers who will be involved in a child's life for only a short time and the positive results may not be apparent until the child is a young adult.

The characteristics of FAS/E make it very difficult for people who have the condition to cope. They frequently end up utilizing a variety of education and treatment resources. Unfortunately, most institutions or agencies have their own philosophical beliefs that are the basis for the form that the intervention or counseling will take. One agency I worked in believed in the family systems approach, and other methods, such as behavior modification, were not allowed. The belief was that if the family members learned how to relate to each other properly, developed adequate boundaries, and the parent's resolved their own leftover childhood issues, then the acting-out child's behaviors would all disappear. In many families this was an appropriate and successful form of therapy, but it was not enough, and not always relevant, with families in which alcohol-related birth defects were present in children. Single-focus approaches seldom work because they are designed for people with problems and needs different from those experienced by children, teens, and adults with FAS/E. The lack of appropriate intervention is partly a result of denial and partially a result of our stubborn refusal to respect the reality and the permanence of the condition.

When we are dealing with a visible handicap, we try to accommodate the needs of the person who is challenged. Yet, with an invisible handicap such as FAS/E, we try to pretend it does not exist, and we deny the alcohol-affected person the right to an appropriate treatment or education. If, however, we are prepared first to acknowledge the condition, second, to involve alcohol affected people in the management of their own condition, and third, to tailor the resources to fit the characteristics, then people with FAS/E will have a much better chance to live normal, successful, and fulfilling lives. To accomplish this, it is important to develop a general understanding of how the individual's life is challenged by the birth defect and to perceive the problems as a whole, rather than as separate problems requiring separate solutions.

The Human Development Framework

The characteristics of FAS/E are so severe and complex that they defy the strict use of any single approach or treatment method. In order to manage the condition on a long term basis, the people involved in the life of an FAS/E child must learn to be versatile and creative and to use different methods for different situations. Fortunately, this does not mean that there cannot be a common basis for developing an effective approach to management. The basis proposed here is the framework provided by the human development process common to all people. It can be used as a jumping off point for both understanding and for managing FAS/E. Human development, when it occurs under optimum conditions, is both predictable and purposeful in that it enhances the individual's capacity to experience a full range of emotions, behaviors, and relationships. The healthy development process allows physiological age, life experience, cognitive skills, and emotional development to move along at a relatively even and congruent pace, so that no particular aspect of the individual's life is stressed beyond the coping ability of the other parts. In other words, the child is able to experience increasing demands on the intellectual and emotional processes with the support of increasing maturation of the body and the brain.

FAS/E interferes with normal development in several ways. First, academic and behavioral disabilities common to FAS/E hold back or confuse some parts of the developmental progress. A low IQ hampers the cognitive development, and while the physical development may be appropriate to the child's age, the emotional part may be years behind. As well, because of the problems with information processing, the child may feel something emotionally, but may not be able to transfer that feeling to intellectual understanding.

Second, developmental progress is a basic human necessity. We are biologically programmed to strive for success in order to stay alive and to master the demands placed on us at each life stage. The characteristics of FAS/E, however, prevent much of that progress so that the individual is left frustrated and unfulfilled and secondary behavioral problems occur.

Over the years, theorists such as Erik Erikson have perceived human development as moving through life stages that have distinct traits.[2] Erikson also suggests that each life stage has a specific task, or goal, and a person's success or failure in achieving that goal will have a strong impact on his or her self-image. If a child is able to meet childhood's goals successfully, self-esteem and self-worth are enhanced. If obstacles prevent success, then negative feelings about *Self* (the child) and *Other* (everyone else) are incorporated into the child's personality.

The stages are seen as occurring in a particular order, with the resolution of one stage necessary before the individual can move on to the next. This does not mean that each stage must be completely resolved before the next is begun, but rather, that the completion of the developmental goals that are part of each stage functions as a base on which the next layer of goals can be assembled. If a child experiences overwhelming obstacles, such as the behavioral characteristics of FAS/E, then a particular stage will be left unresolved. The child is then forced to continue growing physically without the emotional or intellectual resources necessary to cope with the demands of the next life stage.

Helping the individual gain successful resolution of each life stage becomes crucial to the effective management of FAS/E. We cannot get rid of the characteristics of FAS/E, but we can prevent the obstacles from permanently obstructing the developmental process. This is the key to the effective management of the condition. It does not require new skills, or fancy techniques, it simply requires a different way of looking at the behavior.

Notes

1.   R. Dreikkurs, *The challenge of parenthood* (New York: Plume, a division of Penguin Books, 1992) p. 74.

2.   E. H. Erikson, *The life cycle completed* (New York: W. W. Norton & Company, 1982).

Chapter 5
Infancy and Toddlerhood

*I*n the human development model created by Gerald Egan and Michael Cowan it is suggested that the beginning of the developmental stage process occurs in the first two years of life, from infancy to age two.[1] The main goal for all children during this particular life stage is to learn to have a sense of trust in at least two entities. One is *Self* (the infant) and one is *Other* (the parent). As long as the care is regular and appropriate, this new understanding spreads so that infants gradually learn there are many Others, that they are nice, and that it feels good to be with them.

This means that the baby can cry and feel trust that someone will respond and make her feel better. She can develop a sense that there is something beyond herself and that it is good. As well, she can develop positive relationships with other people and learn to trust her own ability to control some aspects of her body and her environment. A simple task such as holding a bottle is a major life event for a nine month old child. It means she can see something she wants, get her little arm to reach for it, and can grasp it and bring it to her mouth. Succeeding at this helps the baby feel good about herself and strengthens her ability to function in the world because she can trust her senses and her skills.

The negative side to trust is mistrust, which develops when the little one cannot predict what is going to happen to her and cannot manage an appropriate level of control over her body and her environment. Babies who receive inconsistent or poor care do not develop an internal feeling of safety in the world. It becomes hard for them to try to reach out to others emotionally, and relationships are a source of instability and insecurity. Because of the total powerlessness of infants, their only solution to bad feelings is emotional withdrawal.

FAS/E can make even simple tasks, like reaching for a bottle, very difficult if there are learning disabilities related to spatial and depth perception. The bottle may almost always appear to be just out of reach no matter how many times she tries. And if she does get hold of it, keeping a grasp on the bottle until it gets to the mouth may be too hard if there are problems with muscle development or coordination. Failure to succeed at such a basic task is not enough to destroy a child's sense of trust, but it is generally part of an overall pattern of failure that is unrecognized by adults and so helps to set the stage for mistrust and the development of an ongoing negative self-image. As the child moves into the early toddler months of life, self-locomotion and the beginnings of speech become central to the child's life. She is biologically predisposed to move and to communicate verbally, yet the unseen problems of poor coordination and speech impediments may become obstacles to her success and may mean that frustration and failure are her constant companions.

Information processing deficit and attention deficit disorder are also present at this early stage and can make it difficult for the child to focus on any of her development tasks long enough to succeed. She can have difficulty tracking what is going on, remembering what she is doing, or following a routine. As a result she may perceive that there is very little predictability to her life even when it is there.

These difficulties can lead to *attachment disorder* and the severe emotional problems that go with that condition. The attachment process in humans was described by John Bowlby as being an instinctive process that occurs when the baby develops a sense of being involved in an emotionally satisfying relationship.[2] The infant first experiences this with its primary caregiver (usually the mother); then the baby expands its ability to relate to include the father, then others such as siblings or grandparents, or baby-sitters.

This process allows the baby to experience the feeling of trust that is so central to successful emotional development at this life stage. As the infant grows older, the positive attachment to the family allows her to feel loved and safe enough to engage in other types of relationships, such as friendships. The teen years allow for attachment to expand to include early attempts at emotional intimacy in the context of a relationship with someone outside of the family, and eventually, the adult form of attachment occurs as a committed and loving relationship between two adults.

As long as healthy attachment took place in the early years, the ongoing process will be based on feelings of self-trust and positive self-image that is expressed on an emotional level as "I am good and I am lovable." The individual will trust her own intuition about others and will pick potential partners who treat him or her as a good, loving, and lovable person.

If neglect or abuse are experienced, or if the FAS/E characteristics prevent the child from experiencing the care and nurturing that could be given, then the attachment process is disrupted and this most primary of relationships is not established. The child is then at risk of growing up without a basic sense of trust and self-worth and may have difficulty forming and maintaining healthy relationships throughout her adult life.

Another way in which the attachment process may be disordered is called traumatic bonding. This occurs when the growing toddler perceives a lack of nurturing or care as life threatening and therefore begins to perceive her own emotional survival as something that is based on the way in which she shows her love for the nonattaching parent. In other words, the little one begins to believe that if she can just love Mommy enough, then she will be all right, and she assumes all of the responsibility for getting the attention she needs. The attention-seeking behavior may take the form of negative acting-out behaviors or the child may become "perfect." Neither method provides emotional health for the child because they both result in her believing that she must accommodate the adult so that she can avoid being emotionally consumed by the terror of emotional abandonment.

As the little one grows up, this traumatic attachment shifts from the parent to other types of relationships. An adult woman who developed a traumatic attachment as a child will stay with a husband who abuses her and their children because she has merely transferred her accommodating behavior from the abusive parent to the abusive husband. She will believe that her emotional survival is based on the relationship and will feel overwhelmed by the fear of abandonment if she tries to leave. Traumatic attachment may also be one reason why some people become cult members. They are seeking to stave off the terror of the early infant abandonment by doing whatever it takes to gain the approval and attention of the cult leader.

Guidelines for Parents and Caregivers

The mainstays of creating successful change for children with FAS/E at this life stage are consistency, routine, and help. *Consistency* should occur in the form of a continuous level of high quality care, the same primary caregiver as much as possible, and in the same surroundings with a minimal number of changes in the environment. *Routine* for alcohol-affected children consists of the days taking on much the same patterns from one day to the next so that the baby can begin to integrate predictability with feelings of safety. *Help* means assisting in the early attempts of the infant or toddler to successfully achieve normal developmental tasks. Consistency, routine, and help facilitate the family's ability to keep the focus during the first months of life on achieving attachment through predictability and touch. Since many alcohol-affected babies may fail to perceive routine and have difficulty with touch, the caregiver has to be as sensitive as possible to the infant's needs. Parents have been rocking babies to sleep since the beginning of time, but for some babies with FAS/E, the rocking motion may be overstimulating, and instead of calming them, it may make them anxious and irritable.

Feeding problems may be reduced by providing frequent, small amounts of nourishment, and they should be given before the baby gets really hungry. If the baby is undereating, it is a good idea to check with the pediatrician to make sure that the baby is getting enough fat and carbohydrates in her diet to make sure that quality is compensating for lack of quantity. As soon as she starts to show signs of hunger, she should be fed, otherwise there is a risk of her becoming too tired or anxious to eat. Each baby displays hunger differently, and the caregiver must learn the signals in order to respond before exhaustion or frustration take over.

The caregiver must also be sensitive to other things that may overstimulate the baby. Many FAS/E babies cannot cope with sights or sounds that other babies generally enjoy. For example, some of these babies are overstimulated by eye-to-eye contact, and others have the same problem with crib mobiles. Seeing what she pulls away from is the best way to tell if the baby is overstimulated. If she does not respond positively to something, take it away. Babies know what feels good and what does not, but they are limited in how they can protect themselves from overstimulation or anything else that is emotionally threatening. Many adults are concerned that they are being manipulated by their babies or children. When infants actually manage to manipulate an adult, however, it is not done to control others, it is done to protect themselves. If they indicate through body language that they do not like something, then there is a reason and the adult caregiver should respond appropriately.

The baby also needs to be touched as much as is reasonably possible. Many alcohol-affected babies cry a lot, which makes them unpleasant to be around. Others are overstimulated by normal cuddling; they actually try to pull away which can make the caregiver pull back as well. Still others have experienced some form of damage to the nervous system that makes touch an uncomfortable or even painful experience. The obstacles to touch must be overcome and most babies will accept some kind of touch if the caregiver is persistent enough to find what is acceptable to each particular infant.

For example, 17-year-old Casey used both cocaine and alcohol extensively until she found out she was three months pregnant. When she knew she was going to have a baby, she became determined to change her life so that the baby "could have it better" than she did. Casey agreed to go into foster care and entered a substance abuse program. After Layla was born, however, it was obvious that a significant amount of damage had been done in those first three months, and one of the worst problems concerned touch. It seemed that any pressure on Layla's skin hurt her terribly and caused her body to go rigid and she would scream for hours. She also suffered from the symptoms of sleep disorder, head banging, and chronic ear infections.

Casey was in a panic about this because she was determined to be a better mother to Layla than her mom had been to her. The social worker had explained about attachment disorder and told Casey that holding her baby would help to avoid it. So, with the tenacity that had helped her survive her own chaotic childhood, Casey kept trying to find a way to touch Layla, and succeeded.

What Casey discovered was that even though the baby's crying was nerve-racking, she could cope with it for a couple of hours at a time if she had the baby in the back carrier. That enabled Layla to feel the warmth of Casey's body without the overstimulation of direct touch. The crying was awful, but the social worker helped Casey to understand that the lonely place inside of Casey herself had something to do with not being touched appropriately or enough when she was little, and she was just going to grit her teeth and do it now for Layla.

Casey also discovered that when Layla was actually asleep, Casey could rub her teeny baby toes without Layla pulling away or waking up. Casey was not sure that this made Layla feel any different, but she knew it made herself feel connected to the baby, so she kept doing it. By the age of three, Layla still had many FAS/E characteristics and Casey was still struggling hard to be a good mother. As a result of Casey's efforts, Layla did not have attachment disorder, and Casey was bonded enough to the child that other problems, such as physical abuse or emotional rejection, did not develop.

Routine and consistency are also important in that they allow the alcohol-affected infant to find anchors in an otherwise confusing world. Keeping the room the same, the crib in the same place, and having one main caregiver are aspects to providing anchors. In today's world, most families try to share infant care between both parents, but the particular needs of the alcohol affected baby may mean that one parent provides as much of the care as she or he can reasonably do. The word *reasonably* is important because all babies are exhausting and FAS/E infants can be more demanding and wearing than others. In these cases, the primary parent simply cannot do it all, but she or he should try to do as much as possible while keeping in mind that this stage does not last forever, even if it seems that way at the time.

As the baby gets older and moves into the toddler stage, she will try to do more, move more, and talk more. Many aspects of daily life begin to be sources of frustration at this age. Trying to build a tower of blocks may be impossible, and holding a spoon so that it goes all the way from the bowl to the mouth may be too great a challenge. At this point, it is important for the parent to step in and help the toddler.

Independence and the process of letting people learn from trying and from making mistakes are experiences highly valued by many people. But if the alcohol-affected toddler is trying and trying to get the spoon to the mouth, cannot seem to do it, and begins to display either frustration or quits trying, then step in and guide the little hand. The baby still gets to do it mostly on her own, the guidance simply assures success.

One of my early mistakes with Jason was to withhold things from him until he said the right word for the object. At the time, I thought I was helping him with his delayed speech problem. For example, when Jason was learning to talk, around the age of 20 months, I would hold a glass of juice in front of him and say "juice," then not give it to him until he said the word back to me. This had worked well with Caryn, she had appeared to enjoy it, and I thought it should work with Jason. What would actually happen, though, was that he would make a couple of attempts, I would think they were not good enough, he would keep trying and failing and I would keep holding the juice in front of him until we both got frustrated and I gave him the juice. I am sure my feelings of frustration wrecked many lunchtimes for Jason and reduced his self-esteem.

Looking back on my behavior at the time, I realize that I would never have been so demanding with Caryn when she was that age. If she made any attempt to say the word, I responded with praise, and if she was feeling stubborn and did not want to talk, I gave her the juice anyway. My worry about Jason's obvious speech delay resulted in unreasonably high expectations on my part, which often became a setup for Jason to fail. As well, my refusal to accept Jason's best attempts was, in effect, a way of punishing him for having the characteristics of FAS/E. It took a long time before I learned the difference between dealing with the behaviors rather than punishing him for having them.

The self-initiative and sense of curiosity that most parents hope to spark in this early stage of life will not be stifled by appropriate handling. The goal is to allow the child to do as much as she can by herself, and step into the situation only when she shows that her self-esteem may be harmed by repeated failure.

Self-Care for Parents and Caregivers

Self-care for the parents must be established very early on in the child's life. The behavioral characteristics cause daily problems that may result in the parents developing a number of confusing feelings or reactions including (1) emotional isolation or withdrawal because the parents feel that nobody else understands what they are going through; (2) the "why me?" syndrome, which can arise when the parents feel both overwhelmed by the difficulties and powerless to change them; (3) angry feelings directed toward the child for having such difficulties and toward themselves for not coping; (4) hopelessness about ever having family times that are normal, fun, and problem-free; and (5) guilt for having these feelings.

These are common, albeit unpleasant, reactions. Many parents of babies or children with this FAS/E are overwhelmed by their own negative feelings yet they keep these feelings a secret out of fear that if they express them to others, they will run the risk of having them confirmed. Parents may be terrified that if others learn the extent of their anger and frustration then others will either judge them as harshly as they judge themselves or may even perceive the parents as incapable of rearing the child.

These are all customary reactions to the ongoing stress of caring for a demanding and needy baby or child. The parents will cope best if they are able to find others in the same situation. Groups that are set up and run by other parents, such as adoptive or foster parent associations, learning disabilities groups, and attention deficit disorder groups can all provide much needed support and agreement for the most negative of feelings. The other members of the organizations can also provide a peer monitoring system, so that parents have support to seek professional help when it is required in order to keep the family functioning.

It is reasonable to try to maintain some kind of life that is not involved with the baby or child. Remembering that the parent is a person with hobbies and interests and skills outside of the parent-baby relationship can help the mom or dad to gain some perspective and to find other means of personal fulfillment. The baby with FAS/E will certainly take up most of the time and energy of the parent, but there must be some time and energy allotted for the parent as an individual and as a marital partner.

I have had many parents tell me that they took regular breaks from the family in order to attend support groups. I encourage them to continue to do so but remind them as well that the purpose of support groups is to focus on the baby. The necessary step beyond that is to attend functions or groups (such as a bowling league or foreign language classes) where nobody cares about your problems at home, they only care about you and your contribution to the activity. This will help the parent to remember that there can still be a place for "fun" and for activities that have no relationship to the problem of alcohol-related birth defects. The point of joining a fun group is that the parent has a place where only she or he, not the child, is important.

The Alcohol-Affected Infant and Foster Care

Infants who are in violent, abusive, or severely neglectful families require child protection services and are frequently placed into foster care. The special needs of the alcohol-affected infant for consistency and routine can pose a real dilemma for foster parents who may only have the child for a short period of time before she or he is either returned to the family or moved on to another home.

Agencies that have a mandate for child protection also have a mandate not to remove children from a home unless there is strong evidence of maltreatment. They are then expected to return children when parents seem to have improved. This is a reflection of society's value to save and protect families, and it serves the best interests of the child in most instances. The special needs of alcohol-affected children involve the consideration, however, that change has the potential to be devastating to the early development of trust, and that minimum levels of acceptable care may not be adequate to prevent attachment disorder. Therefore, a child who has to be removed from a parent may require a longer stay in foster care to ensure that the biological parents are functioning well enough to keep the baby once she is returned. If the baby is subject to frequent change in caregivers she may lose developmental ground and attachment skills with each move. The best interests of the child in this case may dictate that she remain in foster care until the parents have had enough time to display lasting change.

This is not feasible in most areas because judges, who must approve or disapprove the child protection workers' plans, are unfamiliar with matters such as attachment and FAS/E and may not accept a decision to leave a child in care for this type of reason. Parents who understand the problems with FAS/E infants will often cooperate, however, with plans for a longer placement if they know that the ultimate goal is a permanent and successful return of the infant to the parents' care.

The child protection agencies can only try to balance the special needs of the infant with the mandate of the agency. When premature return is dictated, the family will likely require many supports, such as child care workers, in order to successfully manage the baby's special needs. These supports are not available in all areas and resources change from one community to the next. If they are not available, then the foster parent can be assured that the infant will soon be back in care with more damage having accumulated.

Extra supports on a long-term basis are crucial for alcohol-affected infants in families made dysfunctional by alcohol or substance abuse, violence, or severe instability. The type of chaotic environment that is problematic for any child is devastating for FAS/E children. The result of their inability to understand boundaries, limits, rules, and consequences can become life-threatening in the long run if they are in a home that lacks understanding of the condition.

The goal at this life stage is to instill in the baby a sense of safety and trust in Self (who she is) and Other (who everyone else is). The baby should be able to develop a sense that she is a separate being (Self) from those who are around her (Others). Each alcohol-affected baby is different, each family is different, and people can do only as much as their own values, limits, and resources allow. The methods of imparting a sense of trust will vary but the common tools of consistency, routine, and help can be used as guides for anyone caring for a baby with FAS/E. This is not fundamentally different from the requirements of care for any baby. The difference is in the extent of the needs of the baby with FAS/E and the degree of damage that ensues when the needs go unmet.

Notes

1.   G. Egan, & M. Cowan, *People In Systems* (Monterey: Brooks/Cole Publishing Company, 1979) p. 33.

2.   J. Bowlby, *Attachment and loss, vol. one,* (2nd ed.) (New York: Basic Books, Inc., 1982) pp. 38, 47.

Chapter 6
Early Childhood

Early childhood covers ages two to four years.[1] The main goal for this time in life is to develop a strong sense of Self rather than feelings of doubt and shame. A strong sense of Self means that the toddler will know that he is a separate person from those around him, that his ideas and feelings have value, and that his body is his own. He will start to develop an understanding of boundaries and of the difference between what belongs to him and what belongs to others.

The early part of this stage is often called the terrible two's, because it is the time when the little one starts to assert his feelings of ownership and independence by saying no to anything he does not like and perhaps throwing a tantrum when he does not get his way. As frustrating as these behaviors are to most parents, they are vital to the child's burgeoning sense of self-control. Since two-year-olds are too young and inexperienced to do anything right the first time, their version of self-control is usually displayed as an attempt to control everyone else by resisting sharing, not wanting to sleep at bedtime, hating vegetables, and so on. Time and experience teach them to do these things and by the end of this stage they have

59

generally moved past no and are more able to cooperate (at least on occasion).

A sense of Self is difficult to develop when there are obstacles such as attention deficit disorder, poor impulse control, poor short-term memory, and the inability to learn from experience. These characteristics combine to make life unpredictable and chaotic for the alcohol-affected child, as well as making it hard for him to learn any form of self-control. Doubt and shame set in when everything he tries to do gets him into trouble. The normal limits that are provided by caregivers are forgotten before they are learned and normal boundaries simply do not take hold. The child becomes frustrated and stressed by much of his life because his short attention span prevents him from ever feeling that he has accomplished anything.

Parents are also frustrated and exhausted by the behaviors and may start to pull away from the child emotionally. It is not because they do not love him; rather, it is because they see other children progressing and changing through this stage while their four-year-old seems stuck in the terrible two's. And that is exactly what is going on. It is not that the parents are failures, it is that this life stage has far more demands and expectations than the first one and the obstacles presented by FAS/E have a strong impact.

The child can feel his own frustration and sense of failure as well as that of everyone else, and instead of starting to feel good about himself, he starts to feel doubt about everything he tries to do. Since he cannot generalize, he does not know which behaviors will get him into trouble and which will get him cuddled, and he cannot find the link between what he is doing and how people are responding to him.

John Bradshaw, a popular author and speaker on the long-term effects of childhood trauma, suggests that a sense of guilt means that one feels "I did something bad" and that this is a normal part of social control that ensures appropriate behavior.[2] A sense of toxic shame, according to Bradshaw, means that one feels "I am bad" and it results in feeling out of control, worthless, and hopeless. Shame is a terrible emotional burden for someone who is only three or four years old, and it can become an entrenched part of the child's personality. Furthermore, with shame comes despair, also an overwhelming burden to carry on such little shoulders.

Guidelines for Parents and Caregivers

To reach the goal of a strong sense of Self, the tools of consistency, routine, and help remain the most useful for all children. At this stage it is no longer as important that there be one primary caregiver, so long as there is one main set of caregivers that stays the same. In other words, the child may now be able to cope with day care as long as the he or she always returns to the same parents at the end of the day.

It is at this age that children with FAS/E may start to pose a difficulty for siblings. Older siblings may resent the time and energy the alcohol-affected child requires of the parents, and younger siblings may get less than they need for the same reason. It is not possible to reduce the special needs of the child with FAS/E, but it is possible to use supports and services that reduce the demands on the primary caregivers.

Day care on a part-time or full-time basis may be an important part of the family's coping method. The time away from home gives the family a break, and the routine and structure provided in most day care centers and preschools can reinforce the limits and self-control that the child needs to be learning.

For example, Mr. and Mrs. C first adopted Elana, an infant girl from Chile, and seven years later they adopted three-month-old Jarrod through a local public adoption agency. They knew Jarrod's biological mother was an alcoholic and thought they were prepared for FAS/E problems. Jarrod was a challenge from the beginning. Both his eating and sleeping were disordered. He never slept more than four hours at night, and he was always hungry because he would stop eating before he was full. By age two, he was always on the move and his activity level, combined with his lack of impulse control, constantly put his physical safety in jeopardy.

Mrs. C did not work outside of the home and had never considered daycare for either child. She was tired all the time from trying to keep up with Jarrod, but she felt she was managing. When Jarrod was three, the couple adopted another baby, also from Chile. Mrs. C had managed well enough before, but with the new baby, she was just about at the end of her rope. Exhaustion was a constant companion, and both parents found that the added stress was placing their marriage at risk. They decided that they would go against their own values and place Jarrod in day care five mornings a week.

At first that seemed to work fairly well, because Mrs. C was able to have a morning nap with the baby, and the break from Jarrod's demanding needs reduced her overall exhaustion. However, Elana, now age 10 and previously easygoing, began to have tantrums like Jarrod, and every time he walked into the room she would pick a fight with him. Finally, the parents realized that Elana's needs were not being met, and they decided to extend Jarrod's time in day care from nine in the morning to five in the afternoon two days a week. That gave Mrs. C an opportunity to spend a bit more time with Elana after school. As well, Mr. C decided that twice a month he would do something special with Elana on the weekend. It did not have to be any big deal, maybe just the two of them going to McDonald's or going swimming, but it would be their time together.

The guilt they felt over this decision soon gave way to relief, as their family life began to calm down. Jarrod loved day care, the day care staff members were able to cope with him, Elana got the attention she needed, and Mrs. C had more time for Elana and the baby and more energy for Jarrod. The marriage was still a bit rocky, but at least they now had some emotional breathing space and were starting to talk about the problems.

All children at this life stage require constant reminding of rules and limits but most children tend to learn at least enough to give the parents a sense of reward and effectiveness. That is not always the case with alcohol-affected children. These children have great difficulty learning rules and limits and seeing the patterns in life. Since the older they get, the more there is to learn, life for alcohol affected-children and their families becomes increasingly confusing and stressful with each passing year.

The tendency to become involved in parent-child power struggles can begin at this age and can set the stage for major problems in the later teen years. Power struggles give rise to two problems. The first is that no one really wins: the struggle seemingly ends when one of the parties is either worn down and gives up, or one of the parties abuses his or her power to overcome the other. The second problem is that power struggles create a mind-set within the family that the result of conflict is a one-party-win rather than a two-party-resolution.

Power struggles begin when needs or wants conflict. For example, Dad wants Mary to eat her beans and Mary wants to stop eating them. Both Dad and Mary have a right to their own feelings about the beans, but one or both of the parties is going to have to change his or her position. Since the parent is the adult in these situations (a key factor to keep in mind), it is the parent who must decide whether or not the issue is worth pursuing. On the one hand, Mary is entitled to experience power in her own life, so maybe Dad will decide that this is a safe enough issue to let it go. On the other hand, maybe Mary has not yet eaten any of her vegetables and the rule in the family is that nobody leaves the table till dinner is finished, so out of fairness to the siblings, Dad cannot let this one go. Then Dad has to find a way to resolve the conflict. Since food is an area in which the parent can always afford to compromise to some degree, Dad may choose to let her leave after she has eaten one mouthful of beans and vegetables and the next night Dad can make sure that Mary gets a smaller amount of vegetables on the plate in order to avoid a setup of the same problem. If the child is unable to accept the compromise that is being offered, then the father has to use his authority to provide an immediate consequence, such as no dessert. This does not mean that the consequence has to be given with anger or hostility toward Mary, the action alone is enough. There is neither need nor benefit in lectures or long explanations. Dad first tries the compromise, if that does not work then Dad can explain that there is no choice, Mary must eat or face the consequence of no dessert. Ergo, no dessert.

Children with FAS/E have a harder time learning about expectations and limits than many other children, but they will eventually respond to firm boundaries and will learn over time to accept reasonable compromise. It is important, however, that parents remember to allow the child to experience power. Let them win on occasion. Some issues are too important to permit choice or loss, but others can be dropped. Unfortunately, there will be really important issues over which the parents cannot yield control and cannot let go. It is best to save the big battles for the issues where there can be no compromise.

Most parents increase their expectations of the child quite significantly around the ages of three and four. Mothers and fathers who happily picked up the toys at the end of the day generally try to start teaching their child to help with simple cleanup. For the child, however, it is not so simple if he has difficulties with sequencing. For example, asking a four-year-old to pick up his toy truck, take it to his bedroom, and put it in the toy chest is a reasonable request. For an alcohol-affected four year old, however, that task requires that he take in and process a command involving three distinct steps that must take place in a particular order. A child with either an information-processing deficit, sequencing problems, poor short-term memory, lack of impulse control, or attention deficit disorder, is going to find that simple task overwhelming.

A parent can help this child learn how to do a sequence of behaviors by doing them with him. In other words, first the parent tells the child what is wanted, then the parent walks through the task with him. They both go over to the truck so the child can pick it up, they both walk to the bedroom, and they both go over to the toy chest so he can deposit the truck.

This pattern of behavior is another mainstay to effective management. When it comes to cleaning the bedroom, parents can help by breaking the job down into smaller tasks such as picking up the books first, then the little trucks, then the big trucks and so on. The parent will likely have to pick up the first couple of items in each category to give a visual example of what is requested. The parent will also have to help the child understand when each part of the overall task is finished and when to move on to the next. On the negative side, this helping process is complicated and time-consuming, but most young children with FAS/E cannot follow through on requests and sequences without this kind of help. On the positive side, it will ultimately take less time for the parent and child to go through this process than it will take to go through repeated unsuccessful attempts to get the child to cleanup, and the desired outcome will be achieved without anger or failure for both the parent and the child.

The inability to link behavior with consequences also means that there is no such thing as natural consequences. They will, of course occur, but the child will not perceive them as being related to the behavior. For example, if the child purposely breaks a toy out of frustration, the fact that the toy is no longer there to play with will not be a consequence to the child. The toy may be forgotten (out of sight means out of mind), or he may remember that he broke the toy but fails to understand what that has to do with why Mom will not re-place it.

It is important that the parent make the link between the behavior and the natural outcome by verbally stating it. There is, however, no benefit to doing so in a lecturing or yelling manner. Calmly reminding the child that the toy is gone be-cause he broke it is enough, and it can be done any time he initiates the subject. The parent will have to deal with his or her own frustration over the fact that at this age the concept is not likely to have significance to the child. If the parent feels that a consequence is necessary, then create one that has mean-ing to the child. Do not assume that the obvious, natural con-sequence will have any effect.

Organized recreation is popular in North American culture, and children with alcohol-related birth defects can benefit greatly from the opportunity that organized sports provide for devel-oping both social skills and physical coordination. Though these skills are important for the child, the parent will have to assess which activities the child can participate in without disrupting the entire group.

The information-processing deficit, lack of impulse con-trol, attention deficit, and difficulty remembering and learn-ing from experience will make it hard for the child to partici-pate in any group- or team-oriented activities. Trying to un-derstand all of the rules and to act cooperatively, as is required for team activities, may be more than the child can handle. Sports such as swimming and gymnastics are good for muscle development, do not require too much interaction among group members and can be done on an individual basis. The child then has to concentrate only on himself, not on the rest of the team. Choosing an activity at this and in most life stages has a golden rule: if the child likes it and is coping then it is effective, if the child does not like it or is disruptive to other children, pull him out. Time and familiarity do not usually help these children to adjust to situations that have a loose structure or changing rules. The goal of developing a positive sense of Self means that all opportunities must be geared for success. Any that are overstimulating, too unstructured, or beyond the child's skill level, may cause low self-esteem and a sense of shame.

It should be acknowledged yet again that it is also useful for most parents to find a support group of other FAS/E families. Other parents may have helpful ideas for handling a particularly galling behavior, or they may help you to see the humor in a behavior that has pushed you to your limit. Most importantly, support groups give parents a safe and appropriate place in which to express their anger and frustration so that it is not vented on the child.

Most local chapters of special-needs adoptive parents associations or foster parents associations are either offering these kinds of groups currently or are willing to help organize them. In some communities, biological parents are now setting up their own support groups, but in others, the parent groups are made up of all of the different kinds of parents that are involved with the children. If a group does not exist in your community, start one. The support groups in most areas did not exist until a few parents became desperate enough to set one up.

Guidelines for Foster Care, Day Care, and Preschool

In the infancy stage it is important to prevent changes in living situations as much as possible. This approach remains true for the rest of the life stages including early childhood. Each move, even if it is back and forth between the biological parents and the same foster family, creates further delays in the ability to recognize structure and boundaries because the stress of trying to adapt to change may cause the child to lose what he has learned, or to act-out and, therefore, cease to learn until the stress is reduced.

When the child does have to be placed in short-term foster care, it is best (when there is a choice) if he can be the youngest child in the home. Children with FAS/E tend to function at an emotional level that is months or years behind their chronological age, and moving from one home to another may cause traumatic regression. Therefore, placement as the youngest child ensures that they will be treated as such.

Youngsters with alcohol-related birth defects take up as much time and energy in preschool and day care settings as they do at home. Unless there are complicating factors, such as trauma from child abuse, most FAS/E children in this age group can be in a day care center or preschool without any additional staffing requirements as long as the daily routine is structured and predictable and the ratio of teachers to children is high.

Their first few weeks may be a little wearing because they find it difficult to adapt to change, and it will take them a while to perceive the new rules and boundaries. Structure and repetition are key tools in helping the child adjust to the new routine. Structure for these children means that the routine stays much the same everyday, and that the limits and the behavioral expectations are explicit. Repetition of the limits, the expectations, and the routine will, over time, enable the child to begin to perceive the structure. Providing him with the same chair at the same table and facing in the same direction everyday will help to orient him to his new surroundings. Play time also requires structure and routine. It is helpful if the teacher decides what the child should do, as his attention deficit disorder will make it hard for him to initiate and follow through with a task.

Children need a sense of accomplishment, and the poor impulse control and attention deficit disorder will make it hard for most FAS/E children to see anything through from beginning to end. Therefore, the teacher can help by finding short, simple games or tasks that match the child's attention span and by accepting that he is just not going to be able to handle longer activities. One completed task a day is a reasonable goal for the three- or four-year-old. Anything else is likely beyond his abilities at this life stage.

Notes

1. G. Egan, & M. Cowan, *People in systems* (Monterey: Brooks/Cole Publishing Company, 1979) p. 33.

2. J. Bradshaw, stated at personal appearance in Victoria, B.C., 1985.

Chapter 7
Middle Childhood

The next life stage that is common to all children is called middle childhood and comprises the five- to seven-year-old age group. The child's main developmental goal is learning to see herself as an initiator rather than carrying around feelings of doubt about the things she wants or feels. In other words, the child is eager to try new things and is not afraid or ashamed of who she is and how she performs in life.[1]

The overall goal of help or assistance for alcohol-affected children at this stage is to create situations where they can experience success and can have some opportunities to try new experiences, but it is not a good idea to try to deal with everything at once. Decide which problems should be tackled now and which can be ignored for the time being. If parents try to intervene in all of the problem areas at once there will be very little time left for positive interaction between parent and child. As well, the child will end up feeling that there is nothing she can do to please anyone. This kind of attitude can lead to depression at this life stage and acting-out in the teen years.

Praising the child for the things she does well is crucial to her self-esteem, but the praise must be based on things that the child truly does well. Child experts have noted that praise can sometimes create problems if the child begins to doubt the person who is doing the praising, if she does not believe that what is being said about her is true, or if the praise is too general or too lavish.[2] For example, Jason was a poor artist when he was young but like any child, he wanted me to see his pictures and to comment on them. At first I would lie and say they were wonderful, but he stopped that by asking me why I thought the picture was so wonderful when no one else could even tell what it was supposed to be. I then switched from that tactic to doing what I should have been doing from the beginning, which was asking him to tell me about the picture and commenting on the form or the colors instead of the overall picture. I also switched from denying his lack of talent to focusing on if he had fun creating the art and helping him to realize that at his age the point of art class was process rather than product. This enabled me to save praise for the times when it was warranted and he could continue to have faith in my evaluations.

These children hear negative things about themselves all day long so it is important that they hear at least one good thing a day. To keep the praise honest and productive, the parents may have to really search for something, but if we look hard enough, there is always something positive to say. I must be honest, however, and admit that there have been particularly trying days when at the end of them the best I could come up with was to praise Jason for how well he was lying in his bed. This is quite pathetic, but it often creates humor between us and it leaves him going to sleep knowing that I have not given up. I also try to remember to praise my other children every day and not take their relatively good behavior for granted.

If the child knows she has FAS/E, it makes it much easier to engage her in efforts to change the behaviors because an age-appropriate knowledge of the condition can give her a bit of emotional distance from the characteristics. The parents can then approach the need for effective management in a positive way as a joint effort between the adults and the child. This helps the child to feel that she has some control over the problems and is not a continual victim of circumstances. Many of the negative behaviors that result from the frustration of trying to cope with the original characteristics are an outcome of the feelings of hopelessness and confusion that develop when the child does not understand her own condition.

The world greatly expands for this age group as they start school, play with less adult supervision, and become more involved in out-of-home activities. Many of the behavioral characteristics of FAS/E become much more apparent at this life stage as the child tries to make friends and develop sophisticated social and academic skills. Children with FAS/E who have had day care or preschool experience usually find the transition to kindergarten easier than those who have not but it is still a difficult change for them. The size of most schools, the wide variety of rules, and the large numbers of other children can be bewildering.

Most social skills are acquired in subtle, nonverbal ways such as observation of other children, role modeling from adults, experience, and peer pressure. The FAS/E child, however, does not learn this way. Her inability to perceive patterns, to follow through on sequences, to learn from experience and to generalize, means that she may observe what the other children and adults are doing but she will not necessarily understand how any of it relates to her. As a result, she will be slow to pick up age-appropriate social skills and will find that most of what she tries to initiate gets her into trouble. She may begin to hesitate about trying anything new and instead will stick with old behaviors no matter how inappropriate, because at least she can understand how to do them.

To anyone observing the child, the lack of impulse control can make it look as though she never hesitates or stops to think long enough to experience feelings of doubt. And it is true that on a situation-to-situation basis she probably is not feeling any doubt or hesitancy about what she wants. Instead, she develops an overall sense of doubt that acts as a dark shroud over her self-image.

Academic learning disabilities become a concern at this stage. Some of these children have obvious disabilities while others have subtle and fluctuating problems that may not be picked up during the primary school years. It is safer to assume that the difficulties are there rather than waiting until the child starts to fail. Early and repeated neuropsychological testing can give the teachers a reasonable idea of what supports will be needed in the classroom.

Guidelines for Parents and Caregivers

Routine, consistency, and help continue to be the basic tools at this life stage, but parental creativity and adaptability start to play an important role as well. Creativity is the watchword for providing effective discipline, and adaptability is the watchword for learning when and how to use the discipline.

The types of discipline which the parent has experienced as a child or has used with other children may not be effective with the FAS/E child. Different approaches have to be thought of and tried until one is found that works. When an alcohol-affected child consistently and over a period of time fails to respond to an approach, change the approach. Talk to other parents of behaviorally challenged children or to professionals to get some new ideas. Alcohol-affected children are always slow to respond to discipline, but when there is no sign of change then it means that it is not the child who is failing, it is the method of discipline.

Making the consequences relate to the offense is a popular and sensible approach. At this life stage, however, alcohol-affected children still cannot see the links between behavior and consequence, and logical consequences therefore do not exist for the child regardless of how obvious they may be to the parent. It is more important that the consequence of the behavior has an impact on the child than that the consequence be relevant. The first step, therefore, is to help the child understand that negative behaviors have consequences.

Jason used to steal things that he could not possibly use (like drill bits) and hide them in his room. On my regular searches through his room I would find these fascinating items and have to come up with a consequence. One approach that worked well involved having him clean up twigs and small branches that had blown off our the apple trees outside every time I found a missing item in his room. That is a task I would never normally have assigned to a seven-year-old child and it certainly did not relate to what he was stealing. He hated doing it enough, however, for it to have some impact. We never used it as an empty threat: it was put into action the minute I found a stolen item, and we used it only for the length of time that it appeared to slow down his stealing. Like every thing else, it worked only for a few months and I then had to be creative and come up with some other means of discipline for that particular offense.

Whatever the kind of discipline chosen by the parents, it must be immediate, short, and something that the parent is willing to supervise. Unless it happens as soon as the parent sees the negative behavior, the child will not perceive any link between what she has done and the consequence. For example, if she comes home 20 minutes after her curfew, making her come in 20 minutes early the next day will not have any meaning to the child. She simply will not perceive the connection.

The consequence has to be of short duration because she will not likely remember for any length of time why she is being "consequenced" for any length of time. A consequence of long duration may make the parent feel better, but it will not have any impact on the child. Also, the child will naturally resist complying with a punishment, and the short attention span, lack of impulse control and so on, will make it impossible for her to stay on task unless the parent supervises. Therefore, it is in the parents' best interests that the time required for supervision of consequences remain as short as possible.

To increase the effectiveness of consequences, the parents must be sure to follow up on any threats. For example, if Dad and Tommy are shopping at the mall and Dad tells Tommy that any more running up and down the aisles and shouting will result in the two of them going to the car, then Dad will have to follow through the next time Tommy does this. Children with FAS/E do not learn to manage from parental use of idle threats and, like all children, they will cease to listen if they know that parental limits and boundaries are meaningless.

At this life stage, consequences such as time out or removal of toys or privileges may have little impact because what the child with FAS/E cannot see, she cannot remember. If she is grounded to her room, she will forget why she is there, and if her toys are taken away, she will likely forget she had them. The exceptions to this seem to be television and video games. Many alcohol-affected children are quite addicted to these activities and will respond if they are taken away, but over the long run, adding tasks will generally work better than removing pleasures.

The idea of time-out can be adapted, though, so that it is used as an intervention before the child gets into trouble. For example, eight-year-old Dana can play with her friends for about an hour and then things begin to fall apart for her. The interaction between her and her playmates becomes overstimulating and she starts to get exhausted from concentrating on the game. She becomes irritable and bossy and can quickly move into aggression. Dana's mother has learned to check on Dana frequently when she is playing with others and about 45 minutes into a play session her mother will find an excuse to interrupt and change the focus. This may mean providing a snack in the kitchen and having the girls leave their dolls to come and sit at the table for 10 minutes. This type of time-out gives Dana a chance to calm down and prevents emotional eruptions. Her mother also makes sure that Dana has breaks when she is playing on her own because Dana can get as angry at herself as she can at others.

Even when the parents limit the number of issues they focus on, the nagging and consequencing can go on everyday as the behavioral characteristics reach into every area of the child's life. It is important that the parents or caregivers remember to have at least one positive interaction with the child each day. Some days it is easy to be pleasant and feel emotionally close, other days it seems impossible. Without that positive interaction, however, regardless of how forced it may be, the parent and child may start to lose their bond and the foundations of the parent-child relationship may begin to fall apart.

These years can be very difficult as the family and the child adjust to the demands and problems of school. It is easy to place all the attention on the child or children with FAS/E and almost forget nonaffected siblings. They too experience a high degree of stress from the situation. They must cope with having a sibling who steals from them and who frequently embarrasses them in public and yet they often feel an intense need to protect this same person from other children or situations. A nonaffected sibling often becomes trapped in an emotional web that involves being the prime out-of-home protector for the very person that causes him or her to experience the most intense frustration and anger. As well, siblings must cope with parents who are always exhausted and under stress, and the nonaffected siblings are at risk of learning to hide their own problems to protect the parents from having to deal with anything more. They are also at risk of developing acting-out behaviors to get attention for themselves or as a means of escaping from the conflict and stress in the home.

Sometimes the demands of dealing with the child with FAS/E can create a very warped perspective on who is responsible for what. On one occasion, Caryn came to me complaining that Jason had stolen some money from her bedroom and I responded by getting angry at her for failing to lock her bedroom door. Fortunately, Caryn was willing to point out the incongruity of my response. It often takes such an incident, though, to get parental attention directed to the other children.

Almost all of these children have learning disabilities in some or all areas of the brain, making school performance a challenge. Part of the preparation for kindergarten entry should be a complete neuropsychological assessment as well as an assessment by an occupational therapist. Both will give the school system the information required to set up a supportive and effective learning situation in the classroom.

The multitude of learning disabilities that accompany FAS/E are the same as any learning disabilities and require the same educational approach. Any techniques that a special education teacher or teacher's aide might use with other children with learning disabilities will likely be of benefit to the child with FAS/E although the benefits will take much longer to become apparent.

Many parents are able to cope with the hyperactivity during the preschool years but once the child enters the classroom, there is considerable effort to get her to focus and to calm down. The hyperactivity often makes it difficult for the child to learn and in some cases, the child's behavior is so disruptive that the other children are prevented from learning and the child's parents come under increasing pressure to do something to fix the problem. This often means medication such as Ritalin and Dexadrine. This is quite a controversial subject. Some parents, physicians, and teachers see it as the only solution, others believe it results in further damage to the child.

Any decision treating the child's hyperactivity with medication must be made after in-depth consultation between the parents and a pediatrician who knows the child well and has expertise in the use of stimulants for children. There are side effects involved, such as appetite suppression and insomnia, but these negative factors may be outweighed by a lengthened attention span and an increased ability to get through the day. As well, the first medication that is tried may be unsuccessful and the physician may want to try others before finding one that works for a particular child.

There are no medications, however, that will correct all of the problems and the same behavioral approaches will have to be continued. The most that can be hoped for is that a medication that is prescribed will decrease some of the problems and smooth out parts of the child's life. The parents will still have to use routine, structure, and creativity in helping the child learn to manage the FAS/E characteristics and the teacher will still have to deal with a certain amount of behavioral difficulty. If the decision to use medication is made, there must still be a long-term goal of helping the child to learn to manage without pills because it is unlikely that a physician will prescribe medication as a lifelong practice for this type of condition.

Telling the people who are involved in the child's life about the FAS/E condition will usually facilitate their willingness to give that little extra help or attention and therefore increase the child's chance to succeed in a particular setting. Many parents have told me that they do not want other people to know this yet these same people would not hesitate to tell a Brownie leader that their little girl had special dietary needs because of diabetes. Neither condition is within the sole control of the child and neither condition is anything for which the child or parents have to feel ashamed.

The high activity level from the attention deficit disorder persists at this life stage and consequently it is useful to give the child as many energy outlets as possible. Sports such as swimming, skating, and tennis are not luxuries for the alcohol-affected child, they are necessities because they provide a source of stress reduction and build social skills. This is not to say that the child should be involved in activities during all of her waking hours. Sports, if overdone, can be a further source of stress and exhaustion, but most parents can find a balance that works for their child.

Food is another key to managing the high energy level.
FAS/E children burn off a lot of energy, and a regular supply
of healthy sugars (such as fresh fruit snacks) and complex carbohydrates can help the child maintain a degree of attention
and focus in the classroom. As well, FAS/E children often have
finicky appetites, and allowing them to eat frequent, small
amounts of foods can keep them from becoming moody and
uncooperative because of hunger.

Family Foster Care

Foster parents have frequently told me that a child whose
FAS/E includes an IQ low enough to be considered a mental
handicap will have such clear and obvious special-needs that
if she requires family foster care, the foster parents are usually
able to get extra assistance or support services from the placing agency. Unfortunately, if the child has a normal to high IQ
and requires family foster care because of parental neglect or
abuse, the alcohol birth defect may not be diagnosed, and many
of the negative behaviors may be attributed solely to the abuse
experienced in the family.

In such situations, it is commonly thought that placing
the child in a safe environment and providing counseling will
result in changed behaviors. If the child also has undiagnosed
FAS/E, most of the behaviors will remain the same and the
foster parents may find themselves becoming exhausted. It is
not possible for a child protection worker to know if a child
has FAS/E simply by looking for physical characteristics or talking to the parents. If the biological mother has a history of
alcohol abuse it may be reasonable for the foster parents to
request that the child be assessed by a physician who special-
izes in this condition so that appropriate placement plans can
be made.

In almost all cases where a child does have this condition,
the child will require highly skilled foster parents as well as a
counselor or child care worker who can deal with both the
trauma resulting from abuse and the FAS/E characteristics.

Guidelines for Teachers

Teachers often find that children whose diagnosis of FAS/E includes a significantly low IQ can fit into the special-needs categories of school systems because of intellectual impairment. Because FAS/E with a normal or high IQ is not yet well understood, most school districts provide no extra funding for classroom aides or special classes for children with this condition. Often they have been undiagnosed or misdiagnosed as either having solely attention deficit disorder, a learning disability, or a behavioral disorder, and help is either unavailable or inadequate. The classroom teacher is then left with an apparently unteachable child whose negative behaviors prevent the entire class from learning. Even when a diagnosis of FAS/E has been made, the teacher may still be left with the same problems due to budget restrictions that do not allow for adequate classroom support. Some of the same approaches, however, may be used whether the diagnosis is confirmed or suspected because the approaches consist of coping strategies designed to help the teacher get the child through the day in place of changing the curriculum.

Many children with FAS/E find the simple task of entering a classroom overwhelming. Their inability to filter out external and/or internal stimulation means that the normal hustle of the hallway is sheer chaos for them. It is like running through a mine field every morning and the stress can be exhausting. Having the child in question enter the classroom five minutes early is an easy change, allowing the child to begin the day less stimulated and less distracted. This is frequently done for children in wheelchairs and the needs of children with FAS/E are just as valid. The child does not have to be singled out: the teacher can assign four or five students to early entry everyday and no one needs to know it is to get the child with FAS/E into the room.

A teacher suggested to me that this was reinforcing the child's negative behaviors, and the child should just learn to cope. My response was that a child with this condition in this life stage could not simply learn to cope any more than a child with severe muscular dystrophy could simply learn to walk. The goal is to facilitate the child's ability to learn and to behave, but it is a long-term goal and the expectations must be realistic.

Once the child is in the classroom, picture cues can be invaluable. Cartoon drawings of the sequence of expected behaviors can be placed above the coat hanger and on the child's desk. The first set of pictures can show a child taking off her coat and hanging it up, then placing her lunchbox in the appropriate space, then walking to her desk. The picture on the desk can show a child sitting down, facing the appropriate direction, and putting away or getting out whatever supplies or books are required. The picture may be outlined in a bright color so that the child sees it, and it is likely that each week the picture will have to be replaced with a fresh one with a new color so that it does not become part of the unnoticed background.

Many of these children become lost in the process of starting assignments. The teacher gives normal instructions that may include two or more tasks, such as taking out the reading textbook and opening it to a certain page. That simple process involves a sequence and the child will forget the second step. The teacher can assist this process by making sure the student is reminded of the instructions at each step. This may seem time-consuming, but it actually takes less time than sorting out the problems that occur when the rest of the class has begun an assignment and the alcohol-affected child is bouncing around in her seat distracting the other children.

The child will also have difficulty staying focused on the work. Rather than waiting until she is obviously off task, the teacher can intervene every few minutes by using some type of cue to get the child back to work. The teacher and the child can make weekly agreements about what the cue is going to be. It may be a light tap on the shoulder (if the child can cope with touching) or something of that nature. The child will become desensitized to the cue, and it will have to be changed regularly.

I have been asked if this type of intervention does not single out the child with FAS/E and make her problems obvious to the rest of the class. Yes, it does, but it is less humiliating for the child than the kind of singling out that occurs when she is always in trouble and ends up labeled as the class weirdo. One teacher with many years of experience told me that at the beginning of each school year she always has an afternoon where she talks with the children about the different ways that each individual child learns and about some of the conditions, such as learning disabilities, sexual abuse, FAS/E, problems in the home and so on, that can interfere in a child's learning process. She makes it clear that every child is expected to learn and to behave, but that some children in the class may need different kinds of help in order to do so.

This teacher does not single out any of the children or specify who they are. She is well aware that the other children will guess who are the children with special learning and/or behavioral needs, but, as she says, it is better if the class is speculating about learning needs than just assuming these children are dumb or bad. The teacher found that by doing this she was able to provide a more individualized response to those who needed it and the rest of the children were more tolerant and accepting of some of the negative behaviors.

Most of these children will act out in any situation that stresses their ability to cope or to understand. If they are confused about the boundaries or rules, they will misbehave. It can be useful for the teacher to look for patterns of misbehavior that may indicate when a particular activity is too stimulating or confusing for the child. Rules and limits that seem obvious to the rest of the world are often missing for these children. At this life stage, many rules and expectations may have to be retaught everyday.

Learning assistance or placement in a resource room is vital because the basic concepts that the child must learn in these early grades will be forgotten unless the concepts are consistently retaught and reinforced. The degree to which this is necessary cannot likely be done in the regular classroom because it would prevent the rest of the children from making any progress.

At this age, these children may still be overeating or undereating, and they may not have eaten their breakfast or they may have eaten all of their lunch on the way to school. Providing a fresh fruit snack, therefore, around recess and lunch will help keep the children calmer and more focused. If poverty is part of the picture in a school's population, this factor can make it difficult to help an eating-disordered child unless other children are also helped. A principal in an area of high FAS/E and great poverty told me that he had asked a local service club to donate enough money to provide a daily supply of oranges and apples. The teachers in his school, with the help of some parents, took five minutes before recess and after lunch to hand out the fruit and let all of the children in the classrooms have a quick snack. He found that the behavioral improvements were small but were enough that the teachers wanted to continue. And yes, there were occasions of fruit throwing, but they happened less frequently than the eraser and pencil throwing that had occurred before.

The learning environment must also be considered. It helps to place the pupil with FAS/E in the desk or chair nearest the teacher. Close proximity can often allow for fast, proactive intervention. These children do not adapt to a change in routine even when they know beforehand that it is going to take place. Anything that requires a relocation, disruption, or schedule change will likely result in acting-out behavior because the child simply cannot adapt quickly enough. To alcohol-affected children, a change in rules or expectations is the same as the elimination of all rules or expectations. It may be obvious to everyone else that children are expected to behave the same way in the science classroom as they do in the math classroom, but to children with FAS/E, nothing is obvious.

It is important that all tasks and instructions be presented to the child in their smallest components and repeated at least once as the child begins to comply. Multiple directions will be lost due to the sequencing problems. Since the child may not recognize that she is lost or not complying, she is not likely to ask for help or for the teacher to repeat the command. Once the child is working, it will likely take her longer to complete assignments and she will tire very easily from the immense amount of effort it takes her to focus on the work. We often forget that while other children are able to let their subconscious mind do much of the organizational part of the work, the child with FAS/E has to resist the constant urge to move and wiggle, has to actively restrain herself from talking to others, has to remember and work at staying focused on the task at hand, and then has to deal with the learning disabilities that complicate the task.

This process is much like it would be for adults trying to fill out an income tax form that was written in a foreign language, while sitting in the middle of Grand Central Station suffering from an itchy allergy attack. We would never expect ourselves to accomplish such a feat, but children with this condition have to learn to do exactly that every day with every assignment.

Classroom discipline works best if the behavioral expectations and the rules and limits are clearly explained and reexplained regularly and if the consequences for infractions are immediate, short, and consistent. Logical or natural consequences may be as ineffective in the classroom as they are in the home. The point of a consequence is to help the child perceive the structure of the classroom. She cannot "see" the limits the same way the other children do. She must be helped to "feel" them. The consequences are used to enable her to remember the rules, not to punish her for breaking them.

Since children with FAS/E often function at an emotional age that is younger than their chronological age, the child may soon start to seek out younger peers. That is probably going to be a pattern for most of her school life, and if she is in the early grades at school, it may take a while before she is able to make friends. Pairing her up with high functioning peers may be appropriate for some activities but these children do not tend to learn from role-modeling. It is important that the teacher watches to make sure that the child is not feeling overwhelmed and powerless if she is working with the highest functioning child in the class.

Some students may benefit from extra academic support outside of the school, and others may find the day so exhausting that any extra tutoring is useless. The teacher is in an excellent position to let the parents know the child's capacity for additional work. At this age, it is often more important that the child learn to behave in the classroom than it is that she learn to read or do arithmetic. If she is too exhausted from a long day full of expectations, her ability to control her behavior will suffer and even less learning will take place.

The interventions suggested here can make the day and the overall learning process go more smoothly but nothing will make it easy. Children who have FAS/E are hard to teach, and the teaching is time-consuming. Some children may be suffering from the multiple traumas of FAS/E, plus a chaotic home life, plus sexual abuse, plus many moves in and out of foster care. In these cases, it may be that nothing is going to work at that particular time in the child's life. Then, the teacher can only do whatever is possible and not take on a feeling of responsibility for the child's inability to behave or learn at that time. It does not mean that the teacher gives up, or blames the child, rather, it means that the teacher accepts the situation, relates to the child with the most positive attitude possible, and takes whatever normal measures are necessary to ensure that the rest of the class is able to learn.

At one of my recent workshops I met a principal-teacher from Northern Canada who works in a small, remote community that has a high alcoholism rate. She estimates the percentage of children in her school who have FAS/E to be around

75% and she is of the opinion that violence, abuse, and neglect are the norm in most of her students' families. The teachers and the public health nurse provide the only professional services in the area. The nearest physicians, child protection workers, and police are 40 miles away and can be reached only by dirt roads that disappear in the winter. These circumstances combine to make teaching in this school about as difficult as it is likely to get. Rather than fight impossible odds, the principal, early in her assignment to this community, determined the basic needs of the students and set about meeting whatever needs she could. Within six months of her arrival, all of the classrooms in this school had cots placed in the back of the room so that children who had been up all night hiding from violent parents could sleep safely during the day. The principal and the three teachers brought in snacks and sandwiches for the children who had nothing at home, and the main rule of this school was that every child and teen receive a hug or a caring comment at least once a day. This principal has been in the same community for 16 years, she has not burned out, and she continues to update her skills and techniques despite the reality that she may never be able to do more than give these children some safety and perhaps get them to an academic level of about the fifth grade. I think, however, that she is the most successful and effective teacher I have ever met.

Notes

1.   G. Egan, & M. Cowan, *People in systems* (Monterey Brooks/Cole Publishing Company, 1979) p. 33.

2.   A. Faber, & E. Mazlish, *How to talk so kids will listen & How to listen so kids will talk* (New York: Avon Books, 1980) p. 79.

Chapter 8
Late Childhood

The next life stage is late childhood, which includes the 8- to 12-year-olds.[1] The main goal for children in this age group, if they have FAS/E, is to gain a sense of industry, or capability, rather than developing a sense of inferiority. The children still have many of the same needs and problems they had in the previous life stage, but it is at this time that peer relationships start to be a major focus. Social and academic skills take on a new importance, play becomes increasingly complicated and bound by rules. Games provide a forum for group bonding and interaction that gives children an opportunity to develop their interpersonal skills. At this age, children have their first opportunities for unsupervised game-playing, which allows for creativity and spontaneous role-playing.

Children who have FAS/E have a hard time with games and unstructured play because they cannot always meet the social expectations of their peers at this life stage. They seldom remember the rules to the games and as a result are often accused of cheating. Children their own age may shy away from them because they are unpredictable and often in trouble.

Other parents may not want the child in their home because he disobeys the house rules or breaks or steals household items. For the child with FAS/E, this rejection is confusing and hurtful because he does not understand what he is doing wrong.

For example, Shane may know he stole a chocolate bar from his friend's house the last time he was there and a dollar the time before that, but he apologized and promised not to do it again, so it is difficult for Shane to understand why the friend's mother does not want him back. For him, the incidents are over and forgotten. Issues of trust and violation have little if any meaning because he still does not understand personal boundaries. What Shane and others like him do understand is that other kids are always mad at them, teachers are always mad at them, and nothing they try to do works out. School becomes increasingly complex and everyone seems less and less tolerant. They begin to feel inferior and they blame themselves for everything.

The problem with the self-blame is that it is not related to a particular incident and therefore it is not witnessed by others. As a consequence, these children are often mislabeled as "children without a conscience." In fact, they do have a conscience and they feel very guilty about being such a problem, and sometimes they feel guilty about even being alive. However, at the point in time at which others are getting mad, the issues seem confusing and overwhelming to the child with FAS/E and he truly fails to make the connection between the anger and what he has done. He fails to show appropriate guilt at the time because he cannot remember exactly what he did, why he did it, or how it all relates to the present moment. The only honest answer he can usually come up with is "I don't know." Unfortunately, most adults will not accept that and assume it means "I don't care." At this life stage, communication is added to the well-used tools of consistency, routine, help, and creativity. Effective communication skills are a vital necessity in the ongoing success of any parent-child relationship, but they can be overlooked in families who have a child with alcohol-related birth defects. This happens because it is so easy to assign responsibility for all of the problems to the characteristics of FAS/E that other concerns, such as poor communication styles, are ignored.

Effective communication with FAS/E children can be summarized as short, simple, and to the point. FAS/E children often express themselves in this manner and they take in information in the same way. Anything that is longer or more complicated may create confusion or the child may simply tune it out, especially if the child is under pressure or is upset. Normal family dialogue can go on as usual, but instructions, expectations, rules, explanations, and sequenced requests must be short and simple.

In general, the goal of this life stage is to help the child retain his self-confidence and have the courage to keep trying despite the obstacles presented by FAS/E. If he does not succeed at this, he begins to feel inferior to others and becomes vulnerable to depression and secondary behavioral problems.

Guidelines for Parents and Caregivers

It frequently occurs around this age that the child with alcohol-related birth defects begins to become alienated from his peers because of his poor social skills and the learning disabilities that prevent him from following the rules of the group. The fact that the child may have difficulty relating to his peers and being part of a group does not mean that he does not have an inner need to do so. He wants friends and he wants to identify with groups outside of his family just like any other child.

One good thing to do in this life stage is to help the child find activities in which he can succeed and in which he can feel that he is part of a group. If he has already been involved in sports, play groups, or other extracurricular activities, his parent may have a good idea of where the child can fit in. If not, it is time to find something.

Children with FAS/E tend to do better in groups that are structured and have a clear identity. Brownies, Guides, Scouts, martial arts groups, and Navy or Army League often provide the structure, identity, and success that are so crucial to the child. Most group leaders are willing to put extra energy and consideration into working with the child when they know the reasons for the problem behaviors. Leaders then become part of the positive change for the child.

Many parents have told me that they opposed martial arts or military groups because of the violence they represent. I certainly understand that position and, of course, whatever one chooses should fit within the family's values. Most parents of children with FAS/E, however, find that they must make choices and compromises they would never have otherwise considered simply because nothing else works for their child. The main priority is to create alternate opportunities for the child because the normal opportunities have been blocked by the effects of the alcohol. If it works, use it, if it does not work, drop it. If parental values create obstacles to the child's abilities to develop a positive identity, then it may be time to re-evaluate the purpose of those values.

This is the life stage at which the child can start assuming some responsibility for managing the negative behavioral characteristics. The child needs to learn to understand how his behaviors affect others and how his negative behaviors are linked to specific consequences.

Kyle was born to a mother who severely abused drugs and alcohol throughout the pregnancy and who voluntarily placed Kyle in foster care at birth. His mother tried to free herself of substance abuse problems but was not completely successful and by the time Kyle was three years old, it was obvious that he had the behavior symptoms of mild FAS/E. His mother decided to let him be adopted by people who could meet his special needs while she continued to working on her own sobriety.

Mr. and Mrs. F found that they could cope with most of the FAS/E behavioral characteristics but the main problem was that Kyle had a terrible temper. As long as life was smooth and unchanging, he was a sweet and loving little boy who charmed everyone. But the minute things changed, or he could not follow the rules, Kyle started hitting and screaming. His adoptive parents, Mr. and Mrs. F, learned that they could manage his temper in the home by sending him to his room to take some time out or by avoiding situations that made Kyle angry. By the time Kyle was nine, however, he was not always playing in the house, and many of his tantrums occurred at school or in the homes of his few friends. He was quickly developing a reputation as a "mean kid" and peers were beginning to withdraw from him.

One day, Kyle was sent home from a friend's house because the boys had been playing a board game and Kyle, unable to remember the rules, had been accused of cheating. This made him mad and he had thrown the game across the room and hit his friend on the arm. The friend's mother had been very upset and asked Kyle why he had behaved that way. Of course, Kyle had answered "I don't know," which made the parent angry because she thought it indicated stubbornness on Kyle's part. When Kyle got home, his mother gave him some time to cool off, then began tracking with him. This meant that she helped him to recall everything that led up to the outburst. She helped him remember who he was with, what they were playing, what was fun, and when it had stopped being fun. Some of it he could recall and the rest his mother could guess.

Mrs. F explained to Kyle that by being violent, he had failed to manage his anger problem so he had to be "consequenced." The consequence was that he could not go back to his friend's house for three days. She then phoned the other mother, apologized for Kyle's behavior and asked her to let Kyle continue playing there. Mrs. F explained the problems of FAS/E and the other mother agreed to be part of the behavioral change plan. Three days later Kyle went back to play again. The same type of behavior occurred two more times with the same consequence and then Kyle clued in and stopped throwing tantrums at his friend's house. Instead, as soon as he realized he was confused and getting angry, he left the friend's house, went home, and hit his mother on the arm.

Mrs. F's immediate response was to get angry, yell at Kyle, and send him to his room for several hours. She was both shocked and frightened by Kyle's violence toward her and it took two days for her to begin to think about it calmly. She and Mr. F discussed the matter and realized that Kyle had managed to control his anger long enough to transfer it to his mother, but he had not managed to defuse or understand what caused it. Mrs. F went back to basics and sat Kyle down to begin tracking. They started at the beginning of the visit to his friend's, went on to the game to the point where Kyle got angry, left, and went home. She praised Kyle for leaving the scene and then linked his violence toward her with the anger he felt toward his friend. She entrenched the link by giving the same consequence—three days grounding from playing at his friend's house.

The parents were very uncomfortable with Kyle's pattern of violence but they knew he was not yet capable of managing that part of his behavior. They felt that the most they could expect of Kyle at that age was to refocus his rage rather than change it and they bought a punching bag for him. The three of them therefore devised an anger-management plan that involved Kyle taking responsibility for removing himself from the scene when he was angry and directing his violence to an inanimate punching bag. As Kyle gets older, his parents will increase the amount of responsibility they expect from Kyle in anger situations, but right now, they praise him for what he is able to manage.

Tracking is the technique of helping the child recall an event or situation and it can help the child learn to circumvent some of the problems of poor short-term memory. This process involves the parent asking the child to tell the first thing that he remembers of a particular situation and then guiding him on through the memory with relevant questions.

For example, Jason was using the weed cutter to mow down some stubborn grass on our front bank. Two days later I went to use the weed cutter and could not find it anywhere. Jason did not have any recollection of having used it earlier that week. I took him out to the frontyard and asked him which shoes he would normally use to do that chore. He could not remember which shoes he actually wore but he knew which shoes he probably wore so he pictured his feet in those. Then we walked around the bank and I asked him if the day had been hot or cold, if his younger brother had been out there with him at all, and other questions that triggered bits of memory.

Finally, Jason recalled finishing the chore, unplugging the cord, and leaning the weed cutter against a tree on the other side of the property. The tracking was a long process but less time-consuming and less expensive than going out and buying another weed cutter. Furthermore, it helped Jason learn to use his memory without prompting.

It is also important to help the child track through situations that he has managed well. The child with FAS/E is often as baffled about what has gone right as he is about what has gone wrong. Unless the adult helps the child to perceive the successful behavioral choices, he will not likely recognize that he made a choice. Even at this age group, the child sees his life as a series of random, unrelated events.

The parent also has to be consciously looking for appropriate behaviors so that she or he does not lose sight of the fact that they occur. It is very easy for the parent or caregiver to feel so exhausted by everything that the child does wrong, that the things he does right get overlooked. Good behavior is more than an absence of bad behavior and must be given equal attention.

Body Image and Sexuality

During the later part of this life stage, the child may begin to enter puberty. It is vital that children with FAS/E have a solid understanding of how the body works and how it relates to sexuality. They may not recognize potential sexual situations before they happen and so are at high risk of being sexually abused. Many children with FAS/E also behave inappropriately with regard to the physical body aspects of life. They have few boundaries and fail to pick up social cues and they may say or do things that embarrass themselves or others. Very clear do's and don'ts may be necessary to assure that the child behaves in a way that is socially acceptable to his or her peers.

One parent called me to ask what to do about her alcohol-affected daughter, Jillian, who had extremely inappropriate personal habits. This young girl had matured early and was wearing a bra and menstruating earlier than the other children in her class and because of her lack of boundaries she was constantly talking about these things to her classmates. The other children were embarrassed and appalled by the topics and were beginning to call her "weird" and clearly avoiding her as much as possible. To add to the problem, she would forget to wear her bra and some of the children were teasing her badly. Further, Jillian had decided she did not want to menstruate and began to ignore it completely, with dire consequences.

The mother, the teacher, and the school nurse all had long talks with Jillian, explaining everything about the changing needs of a changing body and trying to provide reasons why she had to take better care of her hygiene and why her classmates did not want to hear all about the subject. All of this was to no avail. The problem continued and Jillian was becoming increasingly alienated at school.

It seemed to me that they had tried all the "reasonable" approaches, which had not worked. The only thing left to do was to provide a structure and a routine that left Jillian without choices. I suggested to the mother that she take the responsibility to make sure that Jillian had a bra on every morning and any time she changed clothes. I also suggested that the mother and the teacher keep a diary of Jillian's menstrual cycle and force the issue by making her go to the washroom for hygiene purposes every hour when she was menstruating. They had to hand her the necessary equipment and tell her to go to the washroom. My final suggestion was that every time she started to talk about her body at an inappropriate time, they should simply tell her to stop. Worrying about shutting down the open communication between parent and child was beside the point.

This rigid behavioral approach is not my favorite and goes against my basic values as a parent and a counselor, but it worked for Jillian. After a few months she developed some positive habits about her hygiene, wore her bra all the time, and learned when, and when not, to talk about her body.

It is not uncommon for parents to feel that they lack enough knowledge about sex themselves to be able to teach their children anything useful. In that situation, try to enlist the help of someone else such as a child care counselor or a nurse at the school, or see if there is a group on sexuality at the local YW-YMCA or a church. If no group is available, try to get one started. Again, it is important to look at parental values about sex. One of my clients told me that she did not want her children to know about sex until they were married and had children of their own! I think she was joking, but that is a sentiment shared by many. Unfortunately, it is not realistic and our children are going to be exposed to sex on television, in magazines, at school, and in other children's homes.

The more information the child has, the more choices he can make. Parents also have to make sure that children with

FAS/E understand about the forms of sexuality that may be different from the type practiced in their own homes. They need to know that some teens have premarital sex, that AIDS is a real threat, that some people have abortions, that some are gay, that people masturbate, and all of the other less easy subjects. This can all be taught within the context of the values of each family. Just because a parent does not condone an activity does not imply that the child should not learn about it. Children will be exposed to everything sooner or later (and children with FAS/E are at greater risk of negative forms of exposure such as abuse and exploitation), and they need to have the information that may help them make safe choices. Frank and honest discussions about sexuality at this life stage make it easier to communicate about the same matters when the children are in their more sensitive teens and the realities take on a new level of importance.

Whether or not children with FAS/E are from abusive homes or stable, safe homes, they often place themselves at extreme risk from exploitation by older traumatized children because they cannot relate to their own age group and so seek out the pseudoacceptance provided by the older dysfunctional children or teens. This frequently results in exposure to substance abuse and sexual exploitation. The child or young teen may perceive himself as a willing partner in these activities even though he is, in fact, being abused and exploited. Some of the vulnerable children can avoid this if they receive ongoing support from a child care worker who can help the child understand how he is being used and also help him to find other avenues of friendship and peer identification.

Challenges and Feelings

At this life stage, many challenges confront the child every day. Each day is full of opportunities for failure and stress and the cumulative effect will take its toll on the child. Parents or caregivers can help the child cope with stress in a variety of ways. First, they can acknowledge that it exists and provide emotional support for the child's current stress level. Second, they can give him time off every so often. Sometimes it may help to just keep him home from school for a day so that he can sleep, or let him spend an entire Saturday afternoon playing video games by himself. Third, they can teach him to recognize signs of stress in himself and to help him think of safe and healthy ways of reducing stress. Sniffing glue or other chemical substances is very popular among the 9- to 12-year-old age group. If the parent does not help the child find appropriate means of stress release, other children will.

It should be remembered that children with this condition have a full range of feelings and emotions despite the fact that they may not always display them. They feel compassion and love and concern like everyone else but they may have difficulty expressing complex feelings. For example, my husband, Brian, and I separated when Jason was six but we continued to share the responsibilities of rearing the children and the children were able to maintain a close relationship. Tragically, Brian developed a terminal form of cancer and was very ill for the last few years of his life. Throughout that time, Jason expressed little overt concern or interest in his father's condition. It was not that he did not care but he simply went on with his life as if nothing was really wrong. Part of this was due to his age, part of it was due to the ease with which he could ignore things, and part of it was because he could not conceptualize the fatal outcome of the disease.

A few months before Jason's thirteenth birthday, his father's disease progressed to the final stages and Brian decided to stay in his home and away from hospitals. I tried to help the children understand what was going on but it was impossible for me to judge from Jason's words or behavior just how much he was taking in until one day he told me that he would not be home until supper because he was going to go to his father's after school. I did not know if that was a good idea or not. By then Brian was awake only some of the time due to the heavy doses of medications he was taking to control the pain, but I thought it was not my place to interfere. Brian was still trying to be the best father he could. Because it was too exhausting for him to carry on a conversation, when Jason arrived Brian would get out of his bed and struggle to a chair in the living room so they could watch television together. Brian felt this alleviated the need for conversation and still gave them a way to pass the time together, but it would only be a matter of minutes before he would drift off. When this first happened, Jason was unsure of what to do. There were others around but he did not think to ask them for advice. He knew, however, that he did not want to leave nor did he want to disturb his father. Jason thought about it awhile and then he finally got a blanket and covered his father so that he would not get a chill. Then Jason moved a small chair beside his father's and sat close beside him. This still did not feel like enough to Jason. He reached for one of Brian's hands and held it gently in his own. This became the pattern for their last days together. They would sit in front of the television for several hours at a time, Brian drifting in and out of sleep and Jason sitting beside him holding his hand. We had convinced Jason to go away to a campout that his Cadet group was having over the Father's Day weekend, and while he was gone, his father finally succumbed to the disease. Jason was only 12 and yet in this behavior he displayed compassion, courage, strength, and an ability to give that was far beyond his years.

Respite and Out-of-Home Care

During this age range, it is not uncommon for some of the problems to begin exhausting the parents and the child to the point that they find themselves in continual conflict and too exhausted to use creative methods of change. When this happens, professional counseling is beneficial, but it is not always enough to break some of the ineffectual communication patterns that have developed. It may be that some type of respite care is necessary for everyone to regain emotional strength and learn some new coping methods.

Respite can take the form of having the child go to stay with relatives or close family friends, but the behaviors may be too much for these well-intentioned people as well. It is more realistic that the only situation in which one can find the skills and the willingness to provide respite is professional foster parents. The child may go into a family foster home either every weekend or it may be necessary to use full-time out-of-home care for several months, depending on the severity of the behaviors and the exhaustion level of the parents.

Many parents are terrified of this because they believe it signifies a breakdown of their family. Adoptive parents are often afraid of having their situation considered to be an "adoption breakdown," and biological parents who are already struggling with guilt cannot cope with the thought of feeling further guilt for what may be perceived as a rejection of the child. These feelings have a strong basis in reality because extended family members and professionals may indeed be harsh judges, but the family is more likely to stay together in the long run if they have a well-planned respite than if they continue to struggle until all family members give up.

Over the years I have had many referrals from social workers who were wanting help for a family in which the adopted child was going into out-of-home care with the goal of returning home to the adoptive family within three to six months. Throughout that time, the family and child visited regularly and received weekly family therapy sessions together in my office. These were generally families in which the child had been in the home for anywhere from 8 to 15 years and there was no indication that anyone wanted to terminate the adoption. Yet, time and time again, the contract given to me by the social worker listed the reason for referral as "adoption break-down."

When others around the adoptive family begin defining the problem in these words, what started as nothing more complicated than a family experiencing overwhelming stress somehow gets turned into a failed adoption placement, even if it is 15 years after the adoption took place. The family becomes at risk of perceiving themselves as "breaking down" instead of perceiving themselves as simply requiring some help and a short-term break.

This attitude comes under the umbrella of what Beth Hall and Gail Steinberg have called "adoptism," that is, the "cultural belief that families formed by adoption are less connected than birth families."[2] Adoptive families who live with the stress of FAS/E face the risk of having their problems connected with their status as an adoptive family rather than to their status as a family with an alcohol-affected child.

Biological parents often feel like failures because of prenatal drinking and so perceive any thought of temporary out-of-home care as the final proof that they are "bad" parents. What may happen, though, is that if they continue to struggle to keep the child in the home despite clear evidence that respite is needed, the problems get significantly worse and the feelings of failure and guilt continue to increase anyway.

Families experiencing the stresses and crises that result from living with the pressures of alcohol-related birth defects are not superhuman and cannot become so. It is not unreasonable to expect that there may be times in the child-rearing process in which the stress is overwhelming, the coping methods are failing, and the parents and the child require some time apart. Six months in out-of-home care out of 18 years in the family home is not a failure. It is emotional strength, not parental commitment, that is at issue.

A respite plan that includes short-term out-of-home care placement can allow everyone to relax for a time and recoup their strength. The family can leave doors unlocked, purses and wallets can lie out in the open, and sugar treats can be left in the cupboard. The child can spend some time with people who are prepared to live with the restrictions and who have the skills to help him stabilize if he is feeling out of control. Daily phone contact, regular visits, and family counseling will retain and strengthen the emotional ties.

Communication and Conflict

The strengthening of the emotional ties will also be helped by using a positive communication style. Learning how to listen to what the child is saying, and trying to ensure that both the interests of the parents and the interests of the child are aired will help the child learn how to resolve conflict and will set a positive communication pattern for the later years. Rather than demanding explanations, help the child track what happened. If the information that is being presented is clearly a lie, then state that opinion in a manner that is calm and direct. If the child's hostility level increases, the parents can remind the child that they are not angry and are not yelling. Ask him to take a deep breath, to lower his voice, and to try to hear what is being said. Then, keep the rest short and to the point, without lecturing, blaming, or threats. Just state what is believed to have happened and what the consequence is going to be. If the child is having difficulty controlling his temper, drop the issue of contention for a moment and put all of the focus on helping him to calm down. He may need to go for a quick walk around the yard to let off energy, or he may just need a few quiet moments to let his temper blow over. Once the child is coping again, the parents can go back to the original issue. This process may have to be repeated several times before any resolution occurs, but unless the parent helps the child to learn to communicate in a reasonable and effective way, the original conflict will likely be lost as more and more issues are heaped on top.

Many parents are also lacking in effective communication skills and may have to take a short course or do some reading on the subject to acquire the necessary skills. The parents will have to be discerning consumers of communication techniques; many techniques are too complicated to use with an angry child who has FAS/E. Anything that requires, or is based on, logical thinking will not work. The style that works best is based on a conflict resolution model and assumes that the adult will be responsible for setting a calm, positive tone.

All conflicts cannot be handled well; sometimes everyone will just get angry, and that is all right. There is room in the ongoing parent-child relationship for normal reactions and no parent can be perfect. As long as conflict resolution skills are frequently used, the child will be able to develop them over time, and communication will be open and effective.

Guidelines for Teachers

Teachers will find that all of the guidelines used in previous life stage are still a vital part of assisting alcohol-affected children in the classroom. The child will still likely need to come into the class a few minutes earlier, will still require the picture cues, will still need constant reteaching, and will still benefit from a fruit supplement. Reteaching not only includes going over recently presented concepts, it also means reviewing the basics of arithmetic and spelling.

Routine and structure also remain crucial to the child's ability to get through the school day. Any change in routine represents, for the child, a total loss of boundaries and rules. The class may go to the swimming pool every Friday afternoon for three months and this may appear to be part of the routine to the teacher and the rest of the class. To the child who has FAS/E, however, routine occurs on an hourly, not a weekly basis, and the Friday swim becomes a major change and a loss of familiar structure.

As school becomes more difficult and complex with each passing year, the child may begin to fall behind in some or all subjects. It is often a major task facing these children to simply learn to sit at the desk for a reasonable length of time. Age-appropriate learning goals are not likely to be suitable for the child, and academic goals have to merge with the behavioral goals. During Jason's last year in his elementary school, the main goal was to teach him to work with some degree of independence so that he could adjust to the increased demands of junior high. I think he learned nothing that year in terms of math or science or reading, but he did learn how to cope with less teacher assistance and he was able to manage his behavior well enough that he could concentrate on academic subjects the following year.

Most of the suggestions for teachers that appear in this book were provided by a local learning disability association that is part of a larger nationwide organization.[3] Parents often seek the support and suggestions offered by the local chapters but teachers may not know that these organizations can also provide the same service for school personnel. The suggestions tend to be practical and reasonable and can be used in most classroom settings. For example, the association suggests that the teacher can begin by placing the child near the teacher but away from distractions such as windows or doorways, and helping the student to begin the assigned seat work and then checking back frequently to help him to refocus as necessary. Worksheets can be adapted so that only small amounts of material are on each page and assignments can be broken down into small segments in which the work sequences are separate and clear. Most FAS/E children need a longer time than other students to complete an assignment; the work requirement can be tailored to a length that the student can reasonably be expected to finish. Activities can also be alternated so that some involve standing or moving around the classroom rather than sitting for long periods. Computers, calculators, and tape recorders provide alternate means of helping the child to do the work and often the child's attention span appears to lengthen when he has some kind of electronic instrument to work with. These children often fail tests because they cannot complete them in the given time, or because they are unable to manage the pressure of trying to think and write within a limited time period. Giving the child an opportunity to do tests orally will test the amount of knowledge the child has retained rather than handwriting skill.

Notes

1.   G. Egan, & M. Cowan, *People in systems* (Monterey: Brooks/Cole Publishing Company, Monterey, 1979) p. 33.

2.   B. Hall, & G. Steinberg, "Adoptism—A definition" *Pact Press*, 2(1), p. 18.

3.   Learning Disabilities Association of B.C., South Vancouver Island Chapter, Victoria, B.C., Canada.

Chapter 9
Early Adolescence

The early adolescence life stage, age 13 to 17, represents the years during which the main goal, for most young people, is to learn to associate and identify with the community or else risk experiencing feelings of spiritual and emotional isolation.[1] The young person must go through a process called individuation in which she must learn to detach herself from her family sufficiently to reevaluate her own identity. To successfully identify with the community beyond the family, the youngster must further develop her sense of Self in relation to Other and learn all of the spoken and unspoken rules that will make her acceptable to the community in general. Most youngsters try to identify with segments of the community, such as peer groups, that are not associated with the family. It often seems to the family as though the young teen is doing everything she can to stand out as different from the family, but, in fact, she is probably a carbon copy of the group with whom she is trying to identify.

Parents of 13- or 14-year-olds may complain because their teen has dyed her hair orange, or is smoking, or spends seven hours a day talking to friends on the phone but has not spoken a word at the dinner table in six months. This is the early part of the process of detachment from the family and finding a place in the larger world. It is the beginning attempt to find a place that feels safe and accepting in the larger community.

Many parents question why the teen cannot be like they are, why she has to rebel or emotionally withdraw. The answer is that the parents arrived at their life stage through the same process. It may have taken a different form or a different appearance, but it was the same. The point is that the teen is striving to discover an individual identity and to find a place in which to belong beyond the family. Teens are terrified of being rejected by peers because that is the only form of community available to them at this life stage. It is vital to their development that they find acceptance and become socialized to the larger group.

Most teens have enough social skills to find, through trial and error, a group that is accepting and emotionally safe. The teenager with FAS/E, however, lacks the necessary social skills and may even lose childhood friends when she fails to learn the appropriate social mores. As a result, the teen becomes vulnerable to social isolation. When social isolation occurs, the teen may follow one of two negative paths. The first is to continue trying until she has found a group that is accepting. That group is often one that is involved in high-risk behaviors where drugs, alcohol, and sexual exploitation are the norm. Deaths from drug and alcohol overdoses are not uncommon during these years, nor is estrangement from parents and school. The second path for the teen is emotional withdrawal. Most can cope with this state for only so long and then the buildup of stress and angst sets the stage for some kind of outburst either in the form of violence toward others or suicide.

Teenagers who are progressing successfully through this life stage have generally established some sort of positive association with the community by age 16 or 17, and find a comfortable balance between the expectations of family and friends.

Teens who have failed to establish an identity in the community continue to search and to pull away from the family. Their risky behavior increases in direct relation to their sense of alienation and emotional isolation. Acting-out behavior is not a statement of rebellion, it is a statement of emotional pain.

Jason once said to me that he did not know which parts of his personality were him and which parts were the characteristics of the birth defects. He went on to say that he would never know who he would have been if he had been born free of FAS/E. That was the first time I truly realized what an intense and enormous struggle it is for Jason to find out who he is, and there did not seem to be any response that I could give to ease his confusion or lessen his struggle. I think at that moment, both of us came to realize that Jason was now in a life stage where some of the problems would be too big for me to help him with; that there were now going to be times when the best I would be able to do would be to let him know I cared. That did not feel like enough to me, not after all the years I had spent managing and fixing and rescuing and helping. It still does not feel like enough, but sometimes there are no answers or solutions, sometimes, especially at this life stage, the person with FAS/E has to work through the problems and feelings on his or her own. Parents can provide the supports, but they cannot always do the work.

Guidelines for Parents and Caregivers

One of the most difficult tasks for parents and caregiver throughout the teen years is to learn to distinguish between normal teenage behavior and that which is a result of the FAS/E factor. Many "normal" teens are difficult, moody, rebellious, occasionally rude, forgetful, sloppy, make poor choices, and are generally frustrated and frustrating. It can be hard to learn when to back off and when to intervene. It is a major task for the parents at this life stage to learn to let go so whether it is FAS/E behavior or teen behavior, therefore, the approach may be somewhat the same.

When Jason turned 13, he became very moody. He would get angry with his teachers and me over things that he would have laughed at a year before. I know that anger management is a big issue, so I targeted this as one of the main areas to concentrate on that year. Every time Jason got angry over something, I handled the situation beautifully, which meant I stayed calm, I helped him track his feelings and the events that led to them, I helped him sort out what was rational and what was not, and I then helped him get to a point of stating his problem in a reasonable manner and finding a solution that was suitable to both him and me.

After each episode, I would compliment him on his anger management skills and I would feel like a great parent. My daughter Caryn, however, got angry and asked why I did not treat her as well when she was mad. "When I yell at you, you just yell back," she said, "but when Jason yells at you, you turn into Supermom and take care of him!" She was absolutely right.

There were three things going on here that were not acceptable. The first was as she said, I was not treating her as well as I did Jason. I did not consider that she might also need some parental guidance in order to learn how to handle anger appropriately. The second mistake was in my belief that because Caryn does not have alcohol-related birth defects, I assume that every life stage she goes through is normal and is therefore tolerable. If I find that she is exhibiting behaviors or attitudes that I do not enjoy, I can tolerate them because I know that they are short-term and will be outgrown. But I forget that Jason is also normal in many, many ways, and being crabby and moody is part of being a young teen. He is as entitled to be angry as everyone else, and at this age not every anger situation requires an FAS/E type of intervention.

The third thing I did wrong, in forgetting that Jason is also normal, was to deny him the right to a normal parent-teen conflict. It had been important in his younger years for me to focus on anger-management techniques but he was now at an age where his need to experience individuation meant that some parent-teen conflicts were inevitable. Such conflicts are never fun for either party, but they are a natural part of life and by always intervening instead of simply responding, I was setting up a completely artificial relationship between us. I still use an approach suitable for FAS/E when I see Jason becoming lost in his anger, but the rest of the time I leave it up to his child care counselor to work with him on anger problems and I stick to regular fighting. Even if the teen seems to be coping fairly well, it is a good idea to bring in some extra help at this life stage. A child care worker, a counselor, or someone who has skills relating to teens with FAS/E can help the whole family. With the exception of that mythical teen with the perfect life, most teens must learn to cope with occasional rejection from peers or from members of the opposite sex, and most can benefit from having someone other than the parents with whom they can discuss feelings and sexuality and other sources of confusion. The parents and the siblings may also benefit from having a neutral outside source with whom they can vent their frustrations and discuss ideas.

Rejection by peers often takes place as the teen with alcohol-related birth defects finds it increasingly difficult to keep up with all of the social mores of the group and with the academic expectations of school. Teens who have been lifelong friends may start to pull away from the relationship if the teen is slow to pick up on the unspoken social rules of regular teenage life. As well, the pace of junior and senior high school may become too fast for the teen to keep up either academically or emotionally.

It is also at this life stage that the young person may begin to realize some of the limitations that result from the FAS/E condition. She may still require extensive learning assistance just to get through modified courses while her friends are beginning to compete for the highest grades and to make plans for college. The mother of an 18-year-old once told me that she had always told her daughter, Marcy, that she could do anything as long as she had enough help. The mother did this in order to encourage her daughter and to enable her to keep trying. As the demands of the teen years increased, however, it became apparent that there were many things that Marcy could not do. She could not pass a driver's exam, she could not safely baby-sit children, and she could not keep up with her friends in school. Marcy became very angry with her well-meaning mother and made it clear that she felt she had been lied to. She believed that all of the encouragement was false and that she could no longer trust her parent's evaluations of her abilities. Just as the parent had to grieve in the early years for the lost potential, so will the young teenager experience a sense of loss and grief as she begins to realize the extent and permanence of some of her learning disabilities. Outside services can help her to sort through her feelings and to learn positive coping methods before she becomes at risk for either suicide or acting-out behaviors.

Letting Go

At this life stage, one of the parents' main tasks is to learn how to let go of the control that has been so necessary to help their alcohol-affected child progress through the previous life stages. Once a child reaches her teens, the normal individuation process can take place only if the parents learn to back off and let the teen learn to make mistakes. Letting go is difficult because the kinds of help the child required up to now has meant that the parent was involved in almost every aspect of her life. School, friends, daily schedule, extracurricular activities, have all required intense parental involvement. As well, the intensity of the involvement often means that the parent and the child develop an enmeshed relationship. That is, they spend more time together than most parents and children and they become an overly important part of each other's life.

Nonaffected siblings may also have to learn to let go. It is likely that they have spent many years protecting and helping the sibling with FAS/E and may be as enmeshed as the parents. For example, when we applied to adopt a third child, Caryn was 15 and Jason was 13. The social worker came to interview them individually and one of the questions she asked each of them was why they wanted another child in the home. Caryn's reply was that she wanted another younger sibling because she and Jason had always gotten along really well (we have conflicting memories on this) until Jason became 11 and had acquired enough independence that he no longer needed her. She said that she had felt rejected and hurt by him and she was looking forward to having someone younger again to care for. Although I was concerned about a number of the dynamics involved in this statement, what struck me the most was that I finally understood why she had been so angry with him for the past two years. I had always assumed that it was because he caused her so much stress, and while that was certainly part of it, so was the fact that she had felt rejected and betrayed by his independence. She had gained some of her self-esteem from her role as his protector and helper, and none of us had been prepared to assist her in dealing with her feelings when his need for this role diminished.

This process of letting go of the alcohol-affected youth cannot happen all at once, it occurs over the years with decreasing parental involvement in the areas in which it is safest to hand over control to the teen. This will differ in every family and with every teen and often she will make mistakes and wrong choices. It is safer, however, for her to learn to recover from mistakes at this age than when she is 25.

The most obvious first step in letting go to is to find summer camps that last for at least two weeks. By the time the youngster is 12 or 13, camp should be a regular part of her summer. Some teenagers have difficulty coping when they are away from the familiar routines and rules of home. Most camps, however, will accommodate the special needs of a person with FAS/E as long as the staff members know about it in advance. It is also important that the teen not go to camp at the same time as the nonaffected siblings. This gives everyone a chance to have a break and allows the person with FAS/E to gain some much needed feelings of independence.

The safest areas of responsibility in which parents can begin letting go are in clothing and hair styles. The teen will likely begin using her freedom in this area by choosing anything that the parent will hate, even things like tattoos and body piercing. It is unlikely that any teen has ever died of bad taste or weird hairstyles but it is one of the safer ways to explore individuality and to try different means of self-expression.

The parent or caregiver certainly does not have to condone outrageous clothing, but a parent can state an opinion without getting into a power struggle or a fight. A simple, "I don't really think blue hair works on you, but it is your hair," gets the message across. (I learned this technique from my own mother who said much the same thing to me in response to the hippie fashions of the late 1960s.) Most teens, including those with FAS/E, *want* adult approval but *need* peer acceptance. Learning to control their own appearance is one way to find the balance between the two. Sometimes situations may arise in which the clothing or hair is completely unacceptable. For example, nobody wants a punk in black leather in the wedding photos. If the teen will not cooperate, then leave her out. That is a particularly hard decision for most parents or caregivers to make, but nobody, especially not the parents, wins a power struggle. Just as in the early years of childhood, it is best to save the big battles for the things that really matter.

There have been some occasions with both of our teenagers when the family has been planning an outing that I felt required good clothing and as normal as possible makeup or hair style. When the teen refused to comply, she or he was simply left at home. I did not like those times because the events were important to me, and I was upset that one of the children was left out. But I knew that if I forced the issue, had a fight, and appeared to win because the teen changed his or her clothes to suit me, then my teen would get revenge by being the most miserable and negative person on the planet, and making it impossible for the rest of us to enjoy the occasion. Instead, I pretended to stay calm and said, "Okay, you need to control how you look, I need to not be embarrassed on this occasion, so you don't have to join us." No lectures, no fights, and although nobody won, nobody lost face and the rest of us did enjoy the occasion.

Teens whose appearance is consistently dirty, who do not wash or ever wear clean clothes, or who perform self-abusive acts such using safety pins for nose or nipple piercing, are probably suffering from more than FAS/E. They may have been sexually abused in the past, or they may currently be involved in an exploitative sexual relationship and their appearance has become an expression of emotional trauma. Bizarre behavior or dress could also indicate a wider range of problems such as the beginning stages of a mental illness.[2] If she is dressing like the group in your community that abuses drugs and alcohol, then that is who she is hanging out with and she is likely abusing substances herself. Again, professional counselors or child care workers are invaluable with these types of problems. The family alone cannot help a child or teen resolve external traumas.

Respite and Parental Time-Out

Even for those teens who are not coping with a pregnancy, this is another age during which it may become necessary to place the young person in temporary foster care. In some cases, it may be that the family needs this kind of time out several times over the teen years. As long as there are adequate supports to enable the teen and the parents to continue talking and to stay emotionally connected, then the long-term parent-teen relationship will benefit from the breaks rather than suffer from them.

We hit our emotional breaking point at the same time that Jason reconnected with his maternal biological grandmother. She is a strong woman who appears able to cope with anything; she has become our respite and together we are getting Jason through the last of the teen years. He has grown to love her very much, and the time that he spends with her has greatly helped him to resolve identity issues and to come to terms with his relationship with his biological parents. She is also someone whom I have come to admire and to care about a great deal, and through this contact, our two families have established a large extended family unit.

Parents may want to use respite time to focus on their own relationship and to make sure that it remains stable and healthy for both partners. Years of focusing on the needs of the teen can deplete the richness of any relationship and untended, it can become at risk of dying from lack of attention. Conversely, many marriages become stronger during these years only to break up when this life stage finishes, this happens because the parents become firmly united in parenting but their sole focus has become an end in itself, and is over. Marital counseling or marriage enrichment courses that take place as a preventive measure can help to keep the marriage fresh and alive and can help the couple to remember that there is a life beyond alcohol-related birth defects.

Single parents can use this time to focus on their own needs and priorities apart from the children. If a single parent has found himself or herself too exhausted or broke to have a life outside of the home, now it is time to examine how this happened and to change it. Being a single parent to an FAS/E teenager does not preclude having an active and satisfying social life, nor is it a sentence of loneliness. One single mother, Mrs. L, told me that she could not possibly consider dating while her alcohol-affected teen was still living at home. She felt that it took all of her emotional energy to raise the young boy and that adding the complications of a relationship would be more than she was prepared for. I sympathized with her but reminded her that there were still many nondating social activities such as joining a local gym, taking art classes, learning how to line dance, and so on. Several months later Mrs. L called to say that it had taken a while to find something because of limited finances and limited time, but, she had finally joined a bird watching club and felt that she had found her social niche.

Extracurricular activities for the teen are another area in which the parent must begin to let go. Up to now, the parent or caregiver probably planned every minute of every day in their child's life. But teenagers have to learn to pick their own leisure time activities. The parent might begin the letting-go process by suggesting several sports and letting the teen pick one or two she would like to do. If she is used to lots of out-of-home activity, she will choose to continue to do something, although her need to rebel may mean that, after 10 years of lessons, she quits piano and decides to enroll in gymnastics, which she has never even tried before.

Young teens often earn all of their spending money baby-sitting for other children. It is even a bit of a rite of passage among young teenage girls. Most young people who have FAS/E, however, are not reliable baby-sitters. The same problems of lack of impulse control, inability to link behavior with consequences, short-term memory problems, and so forth, make them ill-equipped to supervise younger children. The teen has to understand her own limitations and must be told the truth about why she is not suitable for the job.

Some alcohol-affected teens may be able to baby-sit, some cannot do so at 14 but can by the age of 16. The parent or caregiver must honestly assess the teen's ability to provide this service and must make sure that the lives of young children are not at risk from one's own child. I have never let Jason baby-sit his younger siblings even for 15 minutes in the afternoon because if he is watching television he focuses totally on the screen and does not notice anything else. It has been suggested to me that I simply tell Jason that he may not watch television when he is baby-sitting. I cannot, however, trust him not to turn it on the minute I am out of the house, so baby-sitting is out of the question. This may change in the future, and I hope it does, but right now it is not possible.

Most teenagers with FAS/E have the same problem with peers at this age as they did when they were younger. It is difficult for them to find a group that will accept them and they attach to almost anyone who will be their friend. If the teen is established in extracurricular activities, she will have a better chance of making friends with other teens involved in the same activities. For example, boys who have no friends at school may have friends in their martial arts group. They may not always be the type of people that the parent would choose as friends for the teen, but the parent and the teen do not really have a choice. The parents can talk with their teen about why they do or do not like the friend, but unless the person is overtly dangerous, allow the friendship to go on and try to supervise it by having the teen invite the friend home as much as possible. Then, at least, the problems engendered by the friendship can be limited and monitored. If there are no friends on the horizon, try to keep the teen busy in as many activities as she can enjoy. For example, when we moved to a new area of town, Jason remained in the same school. He met peers in the new neighborhood, but his social skills were not adequate to establish any new friendships and Jason was miserable from loneliness. We got through this time period by having him attend a local youth club three evenings a week, driving him 30 miles to his Cadet group one night a week, enrolling him in lacrosse, and having his friends from the old neighborhood out on weekends. He did not have a peer group but he was busy, interacting with others his age, and having fun. Eventually, he felt safe enough in one of the groups to begin initiating friendships and he was finally able to establish himself in a peer group. This level of activity is not something I enjoy, and it kept us all busier than we would have liked. But the alternative was for Jason to develop feelings of social and emotional isolation followed by acting out.

Sexuality and Teen Pregnancy

Teenagers with FAS/E begin dating either much sooner or much later than their peers. Unfortunately, neither end of the spectrum appears to be any safer or easier than the other. Because of the lack of boundaries, lack of impulse control, inability to link behaviors to consequences, and the need for acceptance, many of these teenagers date people they do not really like either because they do not know how to say no, or because they are so lonely that they will do anything that appears to give social acceptability.

For all of the reasons just given, dating often leads to overt sexual behavior long before the teen is emotionally or intellectually prepared for it. She ends up feeling guilty, ashamed, and unhappy without really knowing why. She (or he) may assume that because she consented to sexual behavior, she should feel okay about what she is doing. Although the activity may have occurred without coercion, it rarely occurs as the result of informed consent.

The sexual activity may create severe conflict between the teen and the parents and lead to alienation from the family. To keep the teen relatively safe, communication must stay open and honest. Therefore, even though the sexual activity should not be condoned, it also should not be shamed. If the teen has become sexually active she will not initially respond to the parents' approval or disapproval. However, the opportunity to help the youngster out of a bad relationship, or to help prevent pregnancy and disease, will only come about if the teen is not afraid to tell the truth about her life. She cannot ask for help from a parent she is afraid to talk to.

Make sure that the teenager understands the parental attitudes and values, and parents should make clear to the teen when she is veering away from the family's principles. Disapproval can be stated with love, however, rather than with anger. Let her know that even though you do not approve of her behavior, you love her and want her to come to you with problems.

Jason had been dying to have a girlfriend, and in fact, one girl did like him for two weeks and then broke up with him. We all explained that this was normal for his age group and Jason seemed to understand and move beyond the experience, but a few weeks later it became apparent that he had not coped with any of this as well as we had thought.

I was away for four days at workshops in the Queen Charlotte Islands. This is a beautiful area off the coast of northern British Columbia, just below the Alaska Panhandle. The remoteness of the area means that scheduled flights by major airlines are infrequent and I had to remain there longer than I normally stay away from home. On my second night, I phoned home to discover that Jason had not come home the night before. This was quite a shock because he is always 20 minutes late, but he has never failed to show up. It turned out that he had apparently run away to stay with his new love. She was a woman in her late twenties, reputed to have severe emotional problems, alcoholism, and a low IQ. He had since been found by Mrs. G, his best friend's mother, and she had dragged him home.

He was obviously in the midst of great emotional turmoil because he felt that this woman, whom he had met the night before at a local teen hangout, was the love of his life and he just had to be with her. I asked him to stay home until I returned so that we could talk it over in person and I explained to him my concerns that going to live with her would end his schooling, might result in pregnancy or AIDS, and would ruin his future. I also threatened to call the police, but one of his junior lawyer friends had already informed him that 14 is the age of sexual consent where we live so there was nothing I could legally do.

Jason felt that he had a terrible choice to make. He knew all of the risks involved in going back to her house, but his need to be liked, combined with his teenage hormones, was so overwhelming that he could not stay away. All he could finally say was, "But mom, she likes me." Shortly after we talked, he walked out of the house.

There have been many sleepless nights in my life, but this was undoubtedly one of the longest. This situation had never even been one of my worst fears because I had not yet considered that anything like this would happen. I was worried and angry and I was rendered completely powerless by distance and by the situation in general.

Caryn, ever her brother's protector, reassured me that she had tried to talk Jason into staying home but when that did not work, she had packed him a bag of the things she thought he would need. These included a week's worth of clean underwear, a picture of the family, and a package of condoms! I appreciated her levelheadedness, but somehow, knowing that he had these things did not make me feel better.

I got through that night with the help of some kind parents who had raised children with FAS/E and who had spent many nights just like this one. They could not fix anything for me but it sure helped to have people around me who understood not only what I was going through, but also what Jason was experiencing: his loneliness, his need for acceptance at any cost, his need to be what he thought was normal, his desperate need to grasp at someone he perceived to be unconditionally accepting of him. With these people I could talk about what he was doing, and what I was feeling, without any fear of judgment.

I managed to present my workshop the next day and then quickly rushed back to the motel for an update. It turned out that after Jason had left the house, Mrs. G had again gone out and intercepted Jason. She had informed the young woman of Jason's true age (it seems she thought he was much older) and Mrs. G had then taken him to her own house and told him he was staying with them until I returned. This worked well because Jason was happy to be at his best friend's house, was thrilled with all of the attention he was getting, and, I think, was secretly relieved that he had been rescued from his own mistake.

It took a while for Jason to calm down over everything, but he did. He has not been back to that area of town since and has had no contact with the woman. This was typical of the kind of crisis that can happen so quickly with any teens, but especially those with FAS/E. Everything we had taught him went right out of his mind when he was emotionally needy and he had been functioning on impulse and hormones. It was clear, however, that he did not resist being rescued and in fact, has since stated that he was relieved when Mrs. G literally grabbed him by the collar and dragged him into her car. Even if he could not rely on reason, training, or experience at the time, he could rely on adults to take care of him. This intervention was successful because Mrs. G knew he had FAS/E and did not put his behavior down to teen acting-out, and because Jason knows that sometimes he needs help.

Teen pregnancy is reaching epidemic proportions in North America and teens with FAS/E may be more at risk of early pregnancy than others. This is an issue that has a solid impact on the values of each family and different families find different ways of coping with this when it becomes a reality in their home. Some parents may support an abortion while others believe that the pregnancy must be carried to term. At that point, the decision then becomes to place the infant for adoption, to raise the child themselves, to place the child with another family member, or to support the young teen's desire to raise the baby herself.

It is not uncommon, if the teen was adopted herself, that she will have difficulty letting go of her own child, even if she herself is only 13 or 14 at the time of the pregnancy. It is also not uncommon that the teen will follow through with a decision to have an abortion or to place the baby for adoption, but then, when she is unable to cope with her grief, she becomes pregnant again almost immediately. Whatever the decision, if the FAS/E teen decides to become a mother, she will need enormous support to care for the child beginning from the baby's birth and on throughout childhood. Several parents have told me that they found the teen parent coped fairly well while the child was still in its infancy, but could not find ways to deal with the demands of the toddler stage or beyond. Their solution was to either have the teen mom live at home with her baby or to build a suite in their basement or garage so that the parents could provide support and assistance as needed. Clearly, not all parents are in a financial or emotional position to do this, especially over an extended period of time. Nor will all teen mothers agree to such a situation. The local child protective services may have to become involved, but again, that tends to be only a short-term or sporadic intervention. Some teens are able to live in supportive out-of-home care situations with their babies where they receive the kind of valuable support and parenting training that they need. Unfortunately, that ends when the teen mother reaches the age of majority and must then take the baby and try to make it on her own. Tragically, the very teen who is considered too irresponsible to drive a car or baby-sit other people's children, will be left to raise her own child, however inadequate her parenting, because society is failing to provide positive alternatives.

Drugs and Alcohol

Teenagers with alcohol-related birth defects are often exploited by older teens or adults who not only engage the youths in sexual behavior but lead them to drugs, robberies, and/or prostitution. The teen is not likely to stay involved with this type, or even meet them, if she has other areas of social acceptance, but if her social isolation is high, she will be easily victimized.

The usual factors, including lack of impulse control, plus the intense need for peer approval, make the FAS/E teen highly vulnerable to drug and alcohol abuse. The higher a teen's self-esteem, the less likely the youth will abuse illegal substances. The extracurricular activities, parental support, and academic success at any level will help the teen to make healthier choices.

Those teens who do become involved in substance abuse require immediate professional intervention. Parental denial or resistance to involve outsiders will only worsen the problem. Substance abuse treatment for these teens generally takes much longer, sees more relapses, and requires more frequent counseling or group sessions than is provided in standard drug and alcohol treatment. The young person with FAS/E may also resist help or refuse treatment. If that is the case, then the parents and the siblings require help to learn to live with the problem without reinforcing the behaviors. In some instances, that may mean placing the teen in the care of child protective services, or in a residential treatment center, or finding her some other form of living accommodation outside of the home that goes beyond the respite situation.

School, Jobs, and Daily Life

School is an area of severe stress for most teens who have FAS/E. In fact, not all teens can cope with school long enough to graduate while still in this life stage. The emotional struggle and social isolation are so severe for some that the benefits of academic education are negated. Most parents want their child to stay in school and are fearful about what will happen if she does not receive an adequate education. The social and academic pressures, however, are too great for some of these teens. If nothing at school or in the teen's social life is going well, it may be best to remove the youth from school and help her to find some kind of work until she is older and able to cope.

There are all kinds of reentry programs for young people

returning to school, but to be eligible, the youth must be alive and sober. Substance abuse and/or suicidal ideation are often the young person's only perceived method of reducing the stress of social and academic failure. In some cases, it may be necessary to remove the student from the stress before the student removes herself from the world. The parent or caregiver can explain that this is a temporary measure and that the expectation is that the teen will return to some form of education in one or two years. The parent can also explain that this plan is not failure, it is a reasonable alternative to unreasonable stress.

Jobs for teenagers are becoming increasingly scarce as the economy continues to be restructured. Teens who have FAS/E are highly disadvantaged in this aim and will usually require help from parents, friends, or school work placement programs to find part-time or summer work. The purpose of working is not so much one of money as it is of developing independence and increasing self-esteem. Jobs that do not require exchanges of money, use of complicated equipment, or independent activities will more likely lead to success.

Regardless of how good the job looks to begin with, it is always best to prepare the teen for the possibility of being fired. Employers will usually try to accommodate the problems they encounter with employees who have FAS/E, but sometimes they do not have the human resources to provide the necessary supervision, or the problems turn out to be negatively affecting the business. Getting fired is part of the work experience of many teenagers. Let the alcohol-affected teen know that she should do her best and enjoy her work. Let her also know that anyone can have the unpleasant experience of being fired at some time.

If there are no jobs in the area, try to find work projects around the home that can be done for pay. The best projects are those that do not have to get done quickly and that the parents have the time and energy to supervise.

The question of getting a driving license can be contentious in many homes. The alcohol-affected teen may be coping well in many areas of her life, but her impulse control problem may still be too apparent for her to be safe behind the wheel of a car. Do not hesitate to explain this problem to her. It does not help a teen's self-esteem to let her get a license and then make a mistake that costs her own or someone else's life. The decision about when the teen is ready for a license can be made based on her overall behavior and the degree of responsibility she is showing in other areas of her life. Some may be ready at 16, most will not.

Stealing is one of the most frustrating of the behaviors that seem to continue throughout the years, both in an out of the home. Although it is not true in our family, other parents of adults with FAS/E have told me that much of the chronic stealing stops around age 16 or 17. By that time some of the effects of the years of consequences begin to pay off and some of the signs of self-management become apparent. That is, the teen will begin to assume some of the responsibility for managing the characteristics that lead to stealing, such as the lack of impulse control, and to link behavior to consequences.

Until this process takes place, however, parents and caregivers often find that the stealing takes on a new intensity and seriousness once the teen begins to understand what money can buy (i.e., friends, junk food, drugs and alcohol). The amounts of money that are taken become larger than in previous life stages and the frequency of the thefts often increases as well. It is important that the parents not protect the teen from the consequences of theft. Reporting everything to the police is an important part of helping the teen understand that rules, and the enforcement of them, go beyond the family and that consequences can be serious.

In many provinces and states, the laws concerning juveniles make it impossible for the police to provide any kind of meaningful reinforcement of consequences, but having the police pull into the driveway to investigate a theft in the home can have an impact. It certainly has more of an impact than doing nothing. Police involvement combined with strong consequences within the family should at least bring about some reduction in the number of thefts. Consequences should still be immediate, short, and something with which the teen can live.

Because stealing involves a breaking of boundaries and is one of the behaviors that many parents find the most challenging and difficult to cope with, their tendency is to provide a harsh consequence that is designed to make the teen feel as bad as the parent. Consequences that arise from this type of feeling, however, are usually overkill and do not accomplish anything. The point is to provide enough deterrent to make the teen pause and think before stealing again. The point is not to make the young person suffer or to feel unloved. The teenager with this condition does not steal to betray the parents, she steals because she cannot control her impulses and cannot stop to consider the impact of the theft on her victim. Consequences, therefore, are designed to help her place obstacles between her impulses and her behaviors.

All members of the family, including the FAS/E teen, can benefit from a support group. These are hard years during which the family can find themselves under enormous stress. Without the safe outlet provided by support groups, the teenager may become despondent and angry, the other children may begin to act-out, and the marital relationship may suffer. Children and teenagers tend to do best in short term groups of about six to eight weeks duration. Adults do best in groups that are ongoing and permit members to attend on an as need be basis.

Adoptive and foster families usually have access to some type of special-needs adoptive or foster family association that can provide both support and referral. Groups are particularly effective at providing hope, and when it seems that this life stage will never end, there is usually someone in the group who has an older child and can provide assurance and suggestions.

Biological families have more difficulty finding or establishing support groups that specialize in FAS/E because the parents are often ashamed to let people know that they abused drugs or alcohol during pregnancy. But guilt over the past is a poor reason to suffer in the present. When adults show children or teenagers that they are willing to take responsibility for past mistakes, they provide a powerful role model. Also, the fact that a person made a misjudgment years ago does not mean that the person no longer deserves support, respect, and encouragement.

Residential Care and Family Foster Care

Alcohol-affected teens go into residential treatment centers or family foster care for many reasons. Sometimes it is because the home is abusive and the teen is now acting out the resulting trauma; sometimes it is because the parents do not know about FAS/E characteristics, and/or because the parents are simply worn out from years of dealing with the characteristics.

For example, 17-year-old Lindsay had not been diagnosed with FAS/E until she was 16. By that time, she had experienced an unplanned pregnancy, placed the infant for adoption, lived on the streets for a few months on and off, and tried to commit suicide three times. The suicide attempts resulted in brief stays in a local residential facility but placement was of short duration (one week) and follow-up was not mentioned to the parents. After the diagnosis, the parents tried to keep Lindsay at home but she refused to attend school, stayed out for several days at a time, refused to change her clothes or bathe, and kept stealing money from her parents and her siblings. The siblings loved their sister but were embarrassed by her behaviors and hesitated to bring friends home because she stole from them as well. The parents finally decided it was in everyone's best interest if Lindsay could be placed in a treatment center. The only one available for teenagers in their community was a special psychiatric group home for girls that was created to provide long-term treatment for those who had brief stays in the acute treatment center. Since Lindsay had been in the acute treatment center after each suicide attempt, she certainly qualified. The parents did not have to yield custody of Lindsay for her to stay at the group home, and the program was set up for a six-month duration.

The parents, the child protection worker, and the family psychiatrist all met together with the group home staff to provide a history and devise a treatment plan. The parents and the staff members found that they could not agree on the enforcement of limits and rules. The staff members believed it was important that the teen show that she was part of her own healing process by abiding by the curfews and rules. The parents agreed with the principle behind this approach but tried to explain that this must be a long-term goal, not as an immediate expectation. The staff members reluctantly agreed to give Lindsay some time to adjust but were very concerned about the possibility of setting a poor example for the other girls.

Lindsay entered the facility on a Monday morning and, of course, went out that evening and did not return until the next morning. The parents were pleased to hear that she had returned so soon, but the staff members saw this behavior as noncompliance and rebellion and reduced her privileges. This continued for two weeks. The staff members felt they had done what they could without any show of cooperation from Lindsay and she was asked to leave the facility. The staff members said she was unworkable and was not interested in changing. There was nowhere else to place her.

Lindsay went home, disappeared the next day, and is now a prostitute working the circuit. When her parents see her downtown, they take her out and buy her a meal and some warm clothing. They also take her to a clinic to have her various cuts and bruises tended to and can have regular AIDS and pregnancy tests. Neither the parents nor Lindsay ever did anything wrong. They simply did not know what the problem was until she had suffered from years of misdiagnosis and in-

appropriate treatment. By the time they did find out, there
was no appropriate help.

In the optimum type of placement, caregivers will have
clear and consistent rules and limits but will also understand
that the teen may take a year before she is stabilized well
enough to begin obeying them. In the meantime, consequences
must be short, to the point, and not a setup for further failure.
In other words, the consequence must be something that she
can actually do so that she does not end up getting a second
consequence for failing to comply with the first. If that happens, she will lose sight of the original problem, become overwhelmed, and will not be able to make any link between what
she did in the first place and what is happening now. Also, the
facility must be able to commit to providing services to the
teenager for at least two years, because that is how long it is
likely to take a traumatized teen who has FAS/E to stabilize
and to begin working through some of her problems. Anything less will fail to have an impact or bring about change.

One staff member of a group home told me about Robert,
a teenager with FAS/E who had been placed in the group home.
Robert came from a severely abusive background and was not
diagnosed as having this condition until he was 13 and had
received years of inadequate education and inappropriate services. He was a chronic runaway, he abused substances, and
he rarely bathed or changed his clothes. The long-term goals
of the group home staff were that Robert would enter treatment for substance abuse, take counseling for the sexual abuse
he had experienced, and go to school. The initial rules, however, were that he bathe once a week and that he sleep in the
group home one night a week.

After six months they had accomplished those two goals
and added a third, that Robert would eat two evening meals a
week in the group home. The process was slow, but it was
reasonable for what he could actually do at that point in his
life. Recently, I received a phone call from a member of the
group home staff telling me that they were all very excited

because Robert had been found by the police at two o'clock in the morning sleeping in a garbage bin and he had actually asked the officer to phone the group home and have someone come and get him.

When Robert arrived back at the group home, this usually silent teen talked for hours about his life and his feelings. He told them that when he was gone at night he always stayed in that garbage bin because that was where he had hidden from his sexually abusive father throughout his childhood. To Robert, the garbage bin was a place of safety and security. By finally talking about this, he was indicating a readiness to let go of that form of safety and begin to use the safety of the group home. The members of this group home staff were able to see this action as a success and congratulated both him and themselves on the wonderful breakthrough.

Guidelines for Teachers

Teachers will continue to find that the kinds of interventions useful in the previous two life stages remain valuable at the teenage stage as well. Although it is reasonable to expect an increasing level of independence and initiative in classroom functioning and schoolwork from most teens, it is not reasonable to expect such from an alcohol-affected teen until they reach at least 18 or 19 years of age, because their emotional development is usually at least three or four years behind. Teenagers with FAS/E still require consistency, strong academic support services, and patience.

For many teachers, this can be the most frustrating life stage to teach because the teenager has all of the age-appropriate hormones and energy levels but none of the boundaries or social skills that ameliorate the behaviors. Other teens may exhibit an annoying behavior once, get consequenced, and stop, or at least reduce, the behavior. A teenager with alcohol-related birth defects, however, may exhibit a negative behavior in the classroom, receive the consequence, and then turn around and do the same thing five minutes later. This teen will also learn, but she will take four or five times to learn, unlike the learning style of other 14-year-olds.

The curriculum may still have to be adapted to suit the particular learning needs of the student with FAS/E. These teens are often quite articulate and appear to be capable of doing more than they actually are doing. Even at this age, they may still require a regular review of the basics they acquired in elementary school. Material should be presented in parts because the whole may be overwhelming or confusing, and they may have problems understanding the sequence of the work required unless the tasks are presented one at a time. Immediate feedback on assignments is useful because these students may not be able to evaluate their own work. Assignments that relate to real life will help them in their continuing effort to understand how people, ideas, and behaviors connect with each other.

Many teenagers who have FAS/E suffer from emotional problems such as depression, eating disorders, suicidal ideation, and emotional alienation. They may mask their mood disorders with outrageous behaviors, but underneath suffer from loneliness, feelings of worthlessness, peer rejection, and identity confusion.

All of this creates a serious problem if the teen acts these feelings out in the classroom. The behaviors must be dealt with, but so must the underlying feelings. This can best be handled by a school counselor or a referral to a counseling service outside of the school system. Within the classroom, the teacher can deal with the behaviors of these students just as he or she might with any other teen, but with a lower expectation of immediate change and with compassion for the struggle the teenager must endure. It can also be difficult for teachers to cope with the continuing angry outbursts of a teenage boy who is throwing tantrums like a 5-year-old but has the body and strength of an 18-year-old. This presents the classroom teacher with a discipline problem that may involve taking steps to protect his or her own safety, including suspending or expelling the teen if she continues to make others feel threatened by her (or his) outbursts.

If the teen has been diagnosed, the teacher has an opportunity to discuss the problems with the student in the context of FAS/E management. Acknowledging that you, the teacher, understand how hard it is for her, the student with FAS/E, to get though the school day, can do a lot to provide her with the emotional support she needs to keep on trying. As well, if the student understands that the consequences are related to management of the condition, she is more likely to cooperate rather than rebel.

If the student has not been diagnosed, but the teacher believes that the symptoms are consistent with FAS/E, then it is advisable to bring this to the attention of the administration and try to engage the parents in seeking a diagnosis. This kind of discussion with the parents is best done by the vice-principal or a school counselor. If the teacher tries to approach the parents on something of this nature, it could lead to a negative parent-teacher relationship, and neither the student nor the teacher has a chance to improve the situation.

Toward the end of this life stage, the student should begin to take on more of the responsibility for her academic performance and classroom behavior, but this may still be impossible for those with more severe learning or behavioral difficulties or with lower IQ levels. In fact, some students with FAS/E may be unable to initiate action or behave appropriately until their mid-twenties. Therefore, it is important that the teacher perceive the needs and abilities of each student on an individual basis and that the expectations and goals be realistically suited to what the student can, not should, accomplish.

Notes

1.   G. Egan, & M. Cowan, *People in systems* (Monterey: Brooks/Cole Publishing Company, 1979), p. 34.

2.   B. Boulton, M.D., F.R.C.P.C., Victoria, B.C., Canada.

Chapter 10
Late Adolescence

The last life stage to be discussed in this book is called late adolescence and includes ages 17 to 22 years.[1] The chief task facing the young adult at this stage, whether or not he has alcohol-related birth defects, is that of moving out of the home and establishing his own life. This may include beginning a postsecondary education, setting up an apartment, learning to live on a budget, getting a real job, and engaging in serious adult relationships. This is a difficult process for many young people. Most look forward to it with great anticipation because they believe it means freedom of choice, freedom from rules, and an opportunity to be themselves without censorship or monitoring from parents.

The reality is often quite different as they find out that college/university or trade school, jobs, landlords, bill collectors, and so on, all exert far more rules and pressures than parents. As well, they must learn to cope with the new rules and increasing personal expectations with diminishing parental support. Most young adults who do not have alcohol-related birth defects make a number of mistakes in the first part of this life stage but seem to be coping well by the end of it. They are able to see it as a transitional stage from youth to adult and leave it feeling well able to cope with life.

Young adults with FAS/E have a much more difficult time with this transitional stage than others. Many have been undereducated due to their learning disabilities and are not able to go on to higher education or training. In fact, many have not been able to finish high school and do not have the basic language or math skills required for most jobs. Living on their own, and having to budget for monthly expenses such as rent, heat, light, phone, and groceries, are also difficult if they have still not learned to manage money or to understand consequences. They may have learned to baby-sit or do a paper route for money, but prioritizing the living expenses on a limited budget may be overwhelming.

Adult relationships also pose a serious problem. Loneliness, lack of boundaries, and poor judgment lead many of these young adults to make poor choices in partners and to jump into marriage or common-law relationships before they have time to assess the safety and commitment of the potential partner. Although the young adults may not be emotionally or educationally prepared to embark on an independent life, they still have the internal and societal programming that makes them want this. They need to move out, and by this time, the parents or caregivers are exhausted and ready to have them go.

Guidelines for Parents and Caregivers

The help at this stage continues to be a combination of support, encouragement, and letting go. These processes take a much different form than with the previous age group. The young adult who has FAS/E who has managed to finish high school may find entry to further education restricted due to the still existent learning disabilities. At this point, the parent cannot intervene with a simple chat with the teacher and may have to take on the entire institution. Learning disabilities are no less real or valid than physical disabilities, yet they are treated differently by universities and other forms of higher education. Sight-impaired individuals are permitted to use alternate methods of writing exams and using texts but the learning disabled do not always have the same rights. As long as their difficulties will not prevent them from doing the job for which they are training, any means of accomplishing the educational requirements should be acceptable.

Some high schools now help students who have certain designated learning problems make the transition to postsecondary education. These high schools have liaison staff member who, for the first six to eight weeks of the semester, help the new college student to find his classes, organize his workload, set up a study schedule, and work with the instructor to create successful tools for taking notes and completing assignments.

Just as the physically challenged have had to fight for the right to higher education, those with alcohol-related birth defects will have to do the same. If the intellectual level is normal or above, there is no reason why a learning disabled person should not be able to graduate from any university or training program they choose. The institution, however, may not readily agree to this, and the parents may have to help the young adult to challenge this situation through the courts. Discrimination is discrimination, no matter to whom it is directed.

Those adults with FAS/E who could not finish high school at the appropriate life stage may now have the emotional maturity necessary to resume their high school studies and to look into a future beyond that. The time that they took out of school will likely have given them valuable life experience and coping skills that compensate for some of the stress associated with school. As well, the social stresses will be reduced since the young adult will have less need to be part of the "scene" and will have learned more social skills through the work experiences he encountered during his hiatus from high school.

Most young adults start to make plans to move out of the parental home around this time in their lives. The parents and the young adult are often all in agreement that it is time for independence, although it is not always for the same reasons. The parents may be exhausted from the years of stress involved in raising the alcohol-affected person and are happy to let go, and the young adult perceives it as almost a release from bondage. That everyone is looking forward to this life stage, however, does not guarantee success.

The same characteristics of lack of boundaries, inability to handle money, problems getting or keeping a job, and inability to link behavior with consequences (such as spending the rent money on a new television and then being evicted), all combine to make the initial attempts at independence a risky venture. This can be eased if the young adult can first try an alternate living situation that involves room and board or living with some other responsible adult who is willing to help teach budgeting and life skills without taking on a parental role. Some parents have even converted their garage or workshop into a studio apartment as a first step toward independence. If this is not possible, it is best to try for an apartment in the same community as the parents so that they can have regular contact while maintaining separate lives.

The best plan is group homes or other specialized settings for this age group that allow the young adult to move out of foster care or out of the parental home and still live in an environment that provides both monitoring and structure without actual parenting. This would allow the person with FAS/E the extra time he needs to finish growing up while still allowing him to have some of the independence that is desired at this life stage. This type of preparation for an independent lifestyle is rapidly developing in the U.S. out-of-home care system. Some young adults might be ready to leave such a situation relatively soon, others with more severe forms of the condition might require a specialized setting for the rest of their lives.

In any event, if such special support situations are lacking, many of these young people, and the rest of society, pay the tragic costs of their failed attempts at independence. Instead of supporting them in group homes, some are supported in prisons. Some of them cost society nothing, however, because they die from their impulsive behaviors or as the result of the various forms of victimization to which they fall prey.

The parents of less severely alcohol-affected young people may have to be prepared to help their adult child out of the occasional financial bind by paying the rent or some of the other bills. This does not have to become the norm. Helping with money should be concurrent with helping the young adult track the financial or budgeting problems, and it should be done with a clear understanding of the time when this kind of help will end.

This is also an age when many young people begin families of their own. This may occur by planning and choice, or it may happen by lack of planning and accident. People with alcohol-related birth defects who have been raised effectively may be able to raise their own children but at this life stage they would require enormous support to provide adequate care for a child. Unfortunately, persons with FAS/E will often, on an emotional level, continue to function more as a teenager than an adult until the end of this life stage, or, often, until well into the next. The parenting skills may therefore be lacking to the extent that the baby is at risk from the problems associated with the new parents' ongoing difficulty managing their own behavioral characteristics.

The risk that the baby will receive inadequate care is substantially increased if the young mother abused drugs or alcohol during her pregnancy, thereby giving birth to an infant with the special needs caused by alcohol-related birth defects. It is difficult for anyone to meet adequately the needs of an infant with this condition, and it may be impossible for the parent suffering from the same condition without a great deal of support and outside assistance. The grandparents can provide some support in this situation but additional help from public health and social services will often be necessary to ensure that the baby is receiving adequate care. Again, the ideal situation would be a long-term group home for this age group, which could ensure safety for the baby while helping the new mother or father learn how to cope independently.

At the age of 16, Justin was one of the first teens to be diagnosed with FAS/E and many of the necessary supports were added to his education plan and to his life in general. His parents were told that they were lucky because Justin had a normal IQ and he had always had excellent health. The main problems were with the learning and behavioral disorders, but even they were not too severe.

Justin graduated from high school only a year behind his age group but his emotional level remained about three years behind that of a nonaffected 18-year-old, which made it too difficult for him to make the transition to the local community college. He was embarrassed by his failed attempt and refused to try again the following semester. Instead, Justin began to hang around with a group of much younger teens who spent their weekends drinking and their weekdays watching television and playing video games.

Mr. and Mrs. B found this very difficult to cope with. They had worked hard to get Justin through high school, especially in the years before he was diagnosed, and they were afraid that the potential they knew existed within him was going to be lost. Justin was afraid of this too, but he could not face another failure like the one he had experienced at the community college and he found that drinking and playing videos with his new friends helped him to forget his problems.

Mr. and Mrs. B finally told Justin that if he could not get himself a regular job, he could at least start mowing the neighbors' lawns for spending money. This also felt like failure to Justin because it was the same type of menial job he had been doing throughout his childhood and teens. His parents were insistent, however, and when Mr. B put up ads at the local supermarket, Justin knew he had no choice. He began mowing lawns, and built up a large number of customers. This gave

Justin enough money to pay for some of his needs and luxuries, but it was not enough for moving out on his own.

Justin became better and better at mowing. He found he liked being outdoors all day, and he started to take some pride in how the lawns looked after he was finished with them. It also gave him something to do with his time as his drinking buddies drifted away. After a while, the neighbors began to refer him to their friends and also began to ask him to do other things, like trimming hedges and weeding flower beds. Justin complained to his father that he did not know how to do any of this, but Mr. B, instead of providing sympathy, first took Justin to the library to look up pruning and gardening tips, and then enrolled him in a short course in garden care at the same community college Justin had failed at previously. By this time, Justin was almost 23. Many parents would refuse to do so much of the legwork for someone of that age, and many parents would not continue to let someone of that age live at home. Mr. B knew, however, that he could not always expect initiative from someone with alcohol-related birth defects and he took it in his stride to organize parts of his son's life.

The gardening course started the day after Justin turned 23. Much to his surprise, he found that he could keep up with the instructor, and that he even looked forward to going to class. When that course ended, Justin took another, and, with the encouragement of the instructor, he was eventually accepted into a two-year horticulture program. He does not have any real friends, but he works out at a local gym several evenings a week and talks with people there. At this point in time, there are not many signs that he is planning to move out, but because his parents are concerned that he would be lonely and isolated if he were completely on his own, they are thinking of converting the garage into a studio apartment as a halfway step to independence for Justin.

Young adults who received an early diagnosis of FAS/E will find it much easier to establish an independent life than the previous generation because they will have had the opportunity to be adequately educated and supported in their transition to independence. Acknowledging and accepting that he may need additional time to complete high school or to succeed at an independent life will help the alcohol-affected person in this stage to make realistic plans and to accept the supports that the family and community are willing to offer.

Notes

1.   G. Egan, & M. Cowan, *People in systems* (Monterey: Brooks/Cole Publishing Company, 1979) p. 34.

Chapter 11

Conclusion

The characteristics of FAS/E last throughout life and create complications in the lives of the people who have the condition and in the lives of those who live or work with an affected person. The problems associated with the characteristics create numerous secondary problems that can lead to ruined families, ruined relationships, and ruined lives.

None of this is necessary. The condition itself does not have to exist. It is created through maternal, and possibly paternal, alcohol use during pregnancy and can be prevented by abstinence from unhealthy substances. Once the person is born with the condition, it is permanent. The characteristics, however, do not have to ruin lives. They can be managed and the person with alcohol-related birth defects can learn to overcome the obstacles created by the characteristics if she or he has enough of the appropriate services over a long enough period of time.

At this point in history, we barely admit that the condition exists. And, when we do actually recognize the problem, we still tend to deny the affected person the right to be educated and the right to participate in normal social relationships.

Instead, we seek to change and punish the individual for not exerting enough willpower to change his or her brain cells at will.

The truth, however, is that people who have FAS/E can only manage the condition. Any changing to be done must be carried out by those who do not have the condition. The changing must be done by the parents, by the educators, by those who make policy, by those who are friends and neighbors of alcohol-affected persons.

Most children with fetal alcohol syndrome or fetal alcohol effects face more stress, more obstacles, more loneliness, more failure, and less success in a single day than most nonaffected people face in a far longer time. These children are not exceptional because they have the condition, they become exceptional through trying to survive despite all odds. The tragedy lies not in the reality that some people have FAS/E. The tragedy lies in the reality that they are denied their basic human rights to have an appropriate education, to be raised in a supportive environment, and to grow up to be adults who participate in life in a productive and satisfying manner.

Growing knowledge about FAS/E should begin to change this picture, however, and there are fewer excuses for continuing to punish children and adults for problems that are not of their own making. The tragedy can end and the challenge of providing support and appropriate services can begin. The next generation of people with FAS/E should grow up to be educated, taxpaying, productive citizens. They should be able to have satisfying relationships, raise their own children, and earn their own living. There is no longer any reason for the next generation to suffer or die just because their parents made a mistake.

Jason is 18 now. He struggles with all of the normal late teen difficulties and he struggles with the behavioral characteristics of FAS/E. Sometimes he manages very well, sometimes he does not. I keep trying because Jason keeps trying. I try to maintain some perspective on the problems because if I do not, he cannot. I know that Jason does the best he can and that he changes as much about himself as is humanly possible for him. But the amount of change that Jason can accomplish is not enough to get him successfully through life. He cannot do it all. Jason can make himself a more functional person but he cannot make society function better for him. We have to do that. We have to meet Jason and all of the others just like him halfway. They deserve at least that much.

Appendix

Resources

Associations such as those created by adoptive families, foster families, and people with learning disabilities are located in most states and provinces and can provide information on local resources and support groups. The lists below are provided for informational purposes. Inclusion of an organization in this appendix does not constitute endorsement of it by the author or publisher.

Organizations

Canadian Centre on Substance Abuse
75 Albert Street, Suite 300
Ottawa, ON Canada K1P 5E7
613/235–4048
Fax: 613/235–8101
http://www.ccsa.ca/default.htm
email: webmaster@ccsa.ca

Family Empowerment Network (FEN): Support for Families Affected by FAS/E
University of Wisconsin-Madison
519 Lowell
610 Langdon Street
Madison, WI 53703
608/262–8971
Fax: 608/265–2329
Toll Free: 800/462–5254
email: fen@mail.dcs.wisc.edu

FAS/E Support Network of British Columbia

14326 Currie Drive

Surrey, B.C. Canada V3R 8A4

604/589-1854

Fetal Alcohol and Drug Unit

Department of Psychiatry and

Behavioral Sciences

School of Medicine

University of Washington

180 Nickerson, Suite 309

Seattle, WA 98109-9112

206/543-7155

Fetal Alcohol Education Program

Boston University

School of Medicine

1975 Main Street

Concord, MA 01742

617/739-1424

Fax: 617/566-4019

Fetal Alcohol Network (FAN)

158 Rosemont Ave.

Coatesville, PA 19320-3727

Contact: Linda and Hank Will

610/384-1133

Fax: 610/384-6616

email: 72157.564@compuserv.com

Fetal Alcohol Syndrome Family Resource Institute

P.O. Box 2525

Lynwood, WA 98036

206/531-2878

Fax: 206/640-9155

http://www.accessone.com/

~delindam/

email: delindam@accessone.com

NIH/National Institute on Alcohol Abuse and Alcoholism

Office of Scientific Affairs

Scientific Communications

Branch,

Wilco Building, Suite 409

6000 Executive Boulevard

Bethesda, MD 20892-7003

301/443-3860

National Organization on FAS

1819 H Street NW, Suite 750

Washington, DC 20006-3604

202/785-4585

Fax: 202/466-6456

Toll Free: 800/666-6327

http://www.nofas.org/

email: nofas@erols.com

National Resource Center for Special Needs Adoption

16250 Northland Drive

Suite 120

Southfield, MI 48075

810/443-7080

Fax: 810/443-2845, 7099

The Arc
  (The Arc's Fetal Alcohol
  Syndrome Resource and
  Materials Guide)
  National Headquarters
  P.O. Box 1047
  Arlington, Texas 76004
  817/261–6003
  817/277–0553 (TDD)
  http://thearc.org/welcome.html
  email: thearc@metronet.com

The U.S. Department of Health
  and Human Services
  200 Independence Ave., S.W.
  Washington, DC 20201
  202/619–0257
  http://www.dhhs.gov/

The Yukon Association for
  Community Living
  P.O. Box 4853
  Whitehorse, YT Canada Y1A 4N6
  403/667–4606

Books

Alcohol, Pregnancy, and the Developing Child, edited by H. L. Spohr, and H. C. Steinhausen (Cambridge: Cambridge University Press, 1996).

Caring for Children with Fetal Alcohol Syndrome, by Claude Normand, and Deborah Rutman (Victoria, BC: University of Victoria, School of Social Work, 1996).

Children at the Front: A Different View of the War on Alcohol and Drugs, by the CWLA North American Commission on Chemical Dependency and Child Welfare (Washington, DC: CWLA Press, 1992).

Children with Prenatal Alcohol and/or Other Drug Exposure: Weighing the Risks of Adoption, by Susan B. Edelstein (Washington, DC: CWLA Press, 1995).

Crack and Other Addictions: Old Realities and New Challenges, edited by CWLA (Washington, DC: CWLA Press, 1991).

Fantastic Antone Succeeds, edited by Judith Kleinfeld, and Siobhan Westcott (Fairbanks, AK: University of Alaska, 1995).

FAS: A Guide for Families and Communities, by Dr. Anne Streissguth (Baltimore, MD: Brooks Publishing Company, 1997).

*Fetal Alcohol Syndrome/Effects: A
Handbook for Middle-Junior-Senior
High School Teachers,* by Jerry
and Elizabeth Chavez (Washington, DC: NOFAS, 1995).

*Fetal Alcohol Syndrome/Fetal Alcohol
Effects: Strategies for Professionals,*
by Diane Malbin (Center City,
MN: Hazelden Publishing and
Education, 1993).

*Fetal Alcohol Syndrome: From Mecha-
nism to Prevention,* by Ernest
Abel (Boca Raton, FL: CRC
Press, 1996).

*Handle With Care: Helping Children
Prenatally Exposed to Drugs and
Alcohol,* by Sylvia Fernandez
Villarreal, Lora-Ellen McKinney,
and Marcia Quackenbush
(Santa Cruz, CA: ETR Assoc.,
1992).

*Help Me To Help My Child: A
Sourcebook for Parents of Learning
Disabled Children,* by Jill Bloom
(New York: Little, Brown, &
Co., 1991).

*Our Best Hope: Early Intervention
with Prenatally Drug-Exposed
Infants and Their Families,* by
Jane Stump (Washington, DC:
CWLA Press, 1991).

*Understanding the Occurrence of
Secondary Disabilities in Clients
with Fetal Alcohol Syndrome and
Fetal Alcohol Effects: Final Report*
(Seattle, WA: University of
Washington, School of Medi-
cine, Department of Psychiatry
and Behavioral Sciences, 1996).

*When Drug Addicts Have Children:
Reorienting Child Welfare's Response,*
edited by Douglas J. Besharov
(Washington, DC: CWLA Press
and AEI, 1994).

Internet

**AND: The Association for the
Neurologically Disabled of
Canada**
http://www.and.ca/
800/561–1497

Clean Water International
http://www.shadeslanding.com/
clean-water/

**Directory of National Genetic
Voluntary Organizations**
http://medhlp.netusa.net/
agsg/agsgsup.htm

**Family Village: A Global
Community of Disability-
Related Resources**
http://www.familyvillage.wisc.edu/

Fetal Alcohol Related Birth Defects...
http://www.worldprofit.com/
mafas.htm

Fetal Alcohol Syndrome/Fetal Alcohol Effects: A Comprehensive Guide for Educators
http://www.oise.on.ca/
~skalynlangford/fas.html

Fetal Alcohol Syndrome/ Effects Homepage
http://members.aol.com/
jshawdna/fashome.htm

KidsHealth, Org.
http://kidshealth.org/index2.html

National Women's Resource Center
http://www.nwrc.org/
home.html
email: webmaster@nwrc.org

Special Needs Education Network (SNE)
http://www.schoolnet.ca/sne
email: sne@schoolnet.ca
613/526–2200
Fax: 613/526–2703
Toll Free: 800/461–5945

NetStorm Technologies Inc. The Fetal Alcohol Support Network
http://www.acbr.com/fas/
fasmenu.htm

The National Clearinghouse for Alcohol and Drug Information
PrevLine: Prevention Online
http://www.health.org/

About the Author

Brenda McCreight, Ph.D., has a Master's degree in Counselling Psychology from Vermont College, Norwich University, Vermont, and a Doctorate in Human Services from Walden University, Minneapolis, Minnesota. She draws her knowledge not only from personal experience as a biological mother of one child and an adoptive mother of five children (two of whom have FAS/E), but from over 16 years of experience as a therapist working with children, teenagers, and adults with this condition, and from six years of presenting full-day workshops on the topic.

DATE DUE